Praise for *Your Nutritio*

"Sound nutrition advice from a nutrition expert. Filled with practical nutrition tips and tidbits for optimizing gut health, Ms. Tessmer's book is a terrific manual for anyone with or without digestive troubles who is interested in eating their way to optimal health."

—Colleen D. Webb, MS, RDN, CLT

"*Your Nutrition Solution to a Healthy Gut* contains a wealth of information that will improve your gut health, written in an easy to understand and easy to follow format. Kimberly's food lists and suggestions are practical and easy to incorporate into daily living and her nutrition solution tidbits throughout the book help to drive the message home. This is a must read for anyone who has suffered from poor gut health or wants to continue maintaining a healthy gut."

—Lisa Davis, RDN, Clinical Dietitian, Henrico Doctors' Hospital

"Kim has used a basic, easy-to-read and -understand approach to educate the reader on gut health. Her food choices and meal plan suggestions are clearly outlined and easy to follow."

—Johanna Donnenfield, BSc, Phm, MS, RD

your nutrition
SOLUTION
to a
HEALTHY GUT

a meal-based plan to help prevent and
treat constipation, diverticulitis, ulcers,
and other common digestive problems

kimberly a. tessmer, RDN, LD

New Page Books
a division of The Career Press, Inc.
Pompton Plains, N.J.

YOUR NUTRITION SOLUTION TO A HEALTHY GUT
EDITED BY KIRSTEN DALLEY
Cover design by Joanna Williams
Printed in the U.S.A.

To order this title, please call toll-free 1-800-CAREER-1 (NJ and Canada: 201-848-0310) to order using VISA or MasterCard, or for fur-ther infor-mation on books from Career Press.

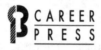

The Career Press, Inc.
220 West Parkway, Unit 12
Pompton Plains, NJ 07444
www.careerpress.com
www.newpagebooks.com

Library of Congress Cataloging-in-Publication Data
Tessmer, Kimberly A.
  Your nutrition solution to a healthy gut : a meal-based plan to help prevent and treat constipation, diverticulitis, ulcers, and other common digestive problems / by Kimberly Tessmer, RDN, LD.
    pages cm
  Includes bibliographical references and index.
  ISBN 978-1-60163-368-2 (paperback) -- ISBN 978-1-60163-384-2 (ebook) 1. Gastrointestinal system--Diseases--Nutritional aspects-Pop-ular works. 2. Gastrointestinal system--Diseases--Diet therapy-Recipes. I. Title.
  RC806.T47 2015
  616.3'30654--dc23

                                        2015010093

disclaimer

At the time this book was written all information in this book was believed by the author to be correct and accurate. Information on gut health changes frequently as more research is being completed. Always keep yourself up-to-date by reading reputable, peer-reviewed, current publications and speaking with your healthcare provider. The author shall have no liability of any kind for damages of any nature, however caused. The author will not accept any responsibility for any omissions, misinterpretations, or misstatements that may exist within this book. The author does not endorse any product or company listed in this book. Always consult with your healthcare provider for medical advice as well as recommendations on any type of drug, supplement, or herbal supplement you plan on taking. The author is not engaged in rendering medical services, and this book should not be construed as medical advice; nor should it take the place of being properly diagnosed and monitored by your regular healthcare provider.

dedication

Dedicated to all of the people who suffer with debilitating gut issues on a daily basis. And to my dear Dad ("Doc") and my late Mom, whom I miss dearly. I have learned so much from them, and continue to learn the power of human compassion from my Dad. I love you both.

acknowledgments

As always, a big, loving thank you to my wonderful husband, Greg, who supports me and works so hard, which allows me to do what I love. And to my beautiful daughter, Tori, who is always patient and understands when Mommy has to work, even if it is at home. I would like to thank all of my fellow RD's who gave me their expert input and advice on this subject. A special thank you to Jan Patenaude, RD, CLT, who is always such a great sounding-board and someone who can always answer my questions. And thank you to all of the dietitians who took time out of their busy schedules to review my book and provide endorsements.

contents

Introduction   15

Chapter 1: Your Questions About Gut Health, Answered   17

What is the gut and what does it do?
What does it mean to have a healthy gut?
What are gut bacteria?
Is there a relationship between certain gut bacteria and disease?
What are the symptoms of an unhealthy gut?
What conditions and diseases are associated with the gut?
Is leaky gut syndrome a real problem?
What are the causes of an unhealthy gut?
How are gut issues treated?
Can a detoxifying diet help my gut?

Chapter 2: The Nutrition Connection and Beyond   47

Our Relationship with Carbohydrates
A Gassy Problem
Uncovering Beneficial Dietary Gut Supplements

Food Allergies, Intolerances, Sensitivities,
and Your Gut
The FODMAP Diet Approach

Chapter 3: Your Five-Step Nutrition and Lifestyle Solution

79

Step 1. Commit to Cleaner Eating
Step 2. Boost Your Daily Fiber Intake
Step 3. Limit Added Sugar
Step 4. Opt for Whole Grains
Step 5. Reach and Maintain a Healthy Weight
Other Gut-Favorable Lifestyle Changes

Chapter 4: 10 Foods to Avoid and 10 Foods to Include for a Healthier Gut

121

10 Foods to Avoid
10 Foods to Include
Gut-Friendly Herbs and Spices

Chapter 5: Menu Planning and Shopping Guide

147

Menu Planning Tips
Navigating the Supermarket
Using Food Labels for a Healthier Gut
Put It All Together
Nutrient Content Claims

Health Claims
Allergan Listings

Chapter 6: 14-Day Menu Guide and Stocking Your Kitchen   181

14-Day Menu Guide
Stocking Your Kitchen

Your Best Resources   209

Bibliography   215

Index   219

About the Author   223

introduction

The term "gut-related disorders" is really just a catchier, more idiomatic name for digestive or gastrointestinal (GI) issues. Gut-related disorders can range from minor to chronic in nature and include all types of health issues, from constipation and peptic ulcers to diverticulitis, just to name a few. Droves of people suffer from these kinds of issues, and because symptoms can be embarrassing, they often refrain from talking about them, sometimes even to their doctor. Instead Americans spend billions of their hard-earned dollars trying to relieve their GI distress by popping over-the-counter medications that are aimed at relieving their symptoms. Though these medications may provide much-needed relief in the short term, they fall short of getting to the root of the problem and treating symptoms over the long term.

Taking preventative steps to ensure a healthier gut can help decrease your risk of developing gut-related disorders, not to mention help manage the ones you might already be dealing with. The gut houses countless numbers of bacteria, some being beneficial and others negatively impacting your health. Choosing the right foods, avoiding the culprits, and adopting healthier lifestyle habits can help to swing the number of favorable bacteria in your favor, thus creating a healthier gut and decreasing your risk for gut-related disorders and their symptoms. The whole idea is not to mask your symptoms with medication but to determine what is causing them and then treating the issue accordingly.

If you suffer from any of the disorders I discuss in this book, you already know first-hand just how downright irritating and uncomfortable they can be. The key is prevention; taking steps now to foster a healthier gut is vital in preventing future issues. This book provides both a treatment and preventative nutritional plan that you can live with for a lifetime. It will guide you by providing useful information in an easy-to-understand format as well as tools to help you modify your diet and your lifestyle in order to help free you from a lifetime of medication, discomfort, pain, and/or long-term health problems. *Now* is the time to take control of your diet and lifestyle to both prevent and manage gut-related disorders. Don't put it off!

chapter 1

your questions about gut health, answered

The phrase "gut health" is becoming a hot topic these days, and there is a valid reason for that. According to the U.S. National Institute of Health, some 60 to 70 million Americans are affected by some type of digestive disease or disorder. And to take it one step further, the health of our gut may not just affect our gut but may affect our overall health. Have you ever heard the phrase "the key to a man's heart is through his stomach"? Well, that might be truer than you realize. The key to better overall health may just be through our digestive tract, including the stomach! In this first chapter we will dive into all of the ins and outs of gut health along with some of the most common GI issues.

What Is the Gut and What Does It Do?

The best way to start is to define exactly what we mean by the gut. Most people think of the gut as the stomach, small intestine, and large intestine (or bowel), but it actually includes much more. In general, "gut" refers to the full gastrointestinal tract, or GI tract. This includes the liver, pancreas, and gallbladder (the solid organs), as well as the mouth, esophagus, stomach, small intestine, and large intestine (the hollow organs). Food starts in the mouth and passes through all of the hollow organs of the GI tract while the solid organs do their part to complete the complex task of digestion. All elements of the digestive system work closely together with parts of the nervous and circulatory systems, hormones, blood, digestive juices and enzymes, and bacteria to thoroughly digest the foods and liquids that we consume each day. The process of digestion breaks down food into nutrients that our body's bloodstream can absorb for needed energy, proper functioning, growth, cell repair, and much more. The small intestine is a valuable asset in this process as it absorbs most of the nutrients, such as vitamin and minerals, as well as water, and then passes them to other parts of the body for use, storage, or further chemical change. What we don't need passes through into the large intestine and exits the body as solid matter, or "stool." Not only does the whole digestive process digest our food and free the body of waste, but it also plays a very important role in protecting the immune system and, therefore, maintaining the health of the entire body.

What Does It Mean to Have a Healthy Gut?

Now that you have a better idea of exactly what your gut is and have a little background on how the digestive tract works, your next question most likely is, "Do I have a healthy gut?" So what does it mean to have a healthy gut? Experts have no technical definition. When it comes to the gut there is no one decisive test that will clue you in as to whether your gut is healthy or not. There are no clear-cut gut tests as there are for other health issues such as heart health, diabetes, or liver function to warn some-one when they are approaching a danger zone. Sometimes knowing whether you have a healthy gut means more of knowing what you don't have. The lack of known diges-tive issues and being able to eat a healthy diet without any resulting GI symptoms such as chronic bloating, gas, heartburn, abdominal pain, and/or constipation can some-times be a sign of a healthy gut. Regular bowel movements and the right amount of beneficial gut flora/bacteria can also indicate a healthy gut. The key is to practice preven-tative measures and keep yourself and your gut in tip-top shape so you have less of a risk of ending up with issues and symptoms down the road.

What Are Gut Bacteria?

It might not sound pleasant but we all have clusters of various strains of bacteria that line the inside of our intestines. In fact, we have hundreds of *trillions* of microorganisms, including thousands of different strains of known bacteria, that live in our gut. Maybe it would sound more pleasant to use the term *gut flora* or, more technically, *gut microbiota*. It is interesting to know that about one-third of the bacteria or gut flora in our gut is common to most people, whereas the other two-thirds is individual to each person. The good news is that the majority of these bacteria is critically necessary and beneficial for our digestive process and our health, so we truly do need them. So the real question is why we need bacteria in our intestines in the first place. The gut microbiota is essential to our health for many reasons, including:

- It helps promote normal gastrointestinal function.
- It helps our body digest certain foods that the stomach and small intestine cannot, such as fiber.
- It helps to regulate metabolism.
- It comprises more than 75 percent of our immune system.
- It helps with the production of vitamins such as B and K. B vitamins are essential for both energy production and the function of the nervous system. Vitamin K is needed for blood clotting and acts as an antioxidant.
- It helps our body to fight against other microorganisms that may not be good for us and provides protection from infection.
- It plays an essential role in strengthening the immune system by creating a barrier effect.

- It helps to produce enzymes that breakdown or digest drugs and hormones and detoxify potentially harmful compounds. In addition it signals the liver to increase production of needed detoxification enzymes.
- It is the key to proper functioning of the digestive system.

Is There a Relationship Between Certain Gut Bacteria and Disease?

Currently researchers are studying the relationship between specific gut flora profiles and health. Current studies are looking at whether certain bacteria might cause disease or whether the opposite is true (that disease might create certain bacteria). Either way, a new approach to looking into a person's individualized gut bacteria may be a way for doctors to more accurately and with greater timeliness diagnose certain diseases. As of this writing, the diseases or conditions that are being studied most intensively in this context are obesity, liver disease, colon cancer, inflammatory bowel disease (IBD), rheumatoid arthritis, certain skin diseases, Crohn's disease, ulcerative colitis, and diabetes. Even though some of these conditions are not gut related per se, gut bacteria are linked to diseases not just of the gut but all over the body. A bacterial imbalance can lead to elevated chronic inflammation, which can lead to health conditions of all kinds. The idea that the gut flora affects general health poses the question of whether we can purposely change our gut flora profile to better our health outcomes. This topic is so important right now that the National Institutes of Health (NIH) recently launched the Human Microbiome Project with more than 100 million dollars to support its research on the effects of gut bacteria on health. Keep an eye out for more concrete results as they become available.

What Are the Symptoms of an Unhealthy Gut?

Symptoms of an unhealthy gut can surface in many different ways. Symptoms can be chronic and may include bloating, gas, diarrhea, nausea, constipation, stomach pain, and stomach cramps. Such symptoms can also be the sign of a specific health condition that has resulted from an unhealthy gut. If you suffer from chronic GI symptoms, you should see your doctor to find out why you are experiencing these symptoms.

Your Nutrition Solution Tidbit: Symptoms of GI health are not always entirely physical. Presenting with some of the symptoms mentioned previously can be very uncomfortable and debilitating and make you downright miserable at times. Gut issues can cause emotional symptoms and stress, as well. When your gut isn't happy, it's hard to be a happy person! Don't be afraid to talk to your doctor about both your physical and emotional symptoms, especially if they are chronic. Talk to your doctor about starting a well-rounded treatment program with all the necessary components, including

diet, weight management, stress management, mental health, exercise, and medication.

What Conditions and Diseases Are Associated With the Gut?

Scientists know that our gut health is directly related to our overall health and vice versa. Certain bacteria that live in the gut are needed to strengthen the immune system; others do quite the opposite and actually promote inflammation. An unhealthy imbalance of these two kinds of bacteria can lead to all types of health problems (not just GI issues), including obesity, allergies, asthma, arthritis, autoimmune diseases, colon cancer, diabetes, and so on. I will discuss some of the more common GI issues in greater detail. Dealing with any of these GI issues can be a sign of poor gut flora or the consequences of an unhealthy gut. It can also be a warning sign of an underlying health issue that is causing the unhealthy gut. For the majority of these issues, following the information and advice in the remainder of this book can help prevent them, or manage them with as little medication as possible.

Peptic ulcer disease

This disease presents as painful ulcers or sores that develop when acid in the digestive tract erodes the inner lining of the esophagus (esophageal ulcers), of the stomach (gastric ulcers), and/or of the upper section of the small intestine (duodenal ulcers). Our digestive tract is coated with a protective layer of mucous that normally will protect against acid from foods and beverages that we eat as well as from the acid that our stomach produces naturally. We need some acid in our digestive tract for normal digestion and breakdown of foods. However, if the amount of acid is increased or the amount of mucous is decreased, an ulcer may develop.

Several different factors can affect gut health and the balance of gastric acid, thus increasing your chances of or causing ulcers. A major factor is a specific bacterium known as *Helicobacter pylori* (*H. pylori*) is able to penetrate the protective mucous lining of the stomach, where it produces substances that weaken the lining and make the stomach more susceptible to peptic ulcers. Scientists are not completely sure how *H. pylori* spreads, but have theorized that it is transmitted from person to person by close contact and/or through infected food and water. *H. pylori* can be a major cause of chronic gastritis and peptic ulcers, and can increase your risk for stomach cancer.

Over-the-counter and prescription painkillers, especially in older adults and those who overuse them, can also be factors. Nonsteroidal anti-inflammatory drugs (NSAIDs) in particular, including aspirin, naproxen, and ibuprofen, can irritate and inflame the inner lining of the stomach and small intestine. Some prescription medications, such as Fosamax, Actonel, and even some potassium supplements, can lead to ulcers and should be used only under close supervision by a doctor.

Other factors:

- Excess acid production within the GI system.
- Excessive intake of alcohol.

- Smoking and chewing tobacco.

- Family history of peptic ulcers and/or personal history of previous ulcers.

- Being more than 50 years old.

- Serious illness such as stomach cancer and liver or kidney disease.

- Radiation treatment to the GI area.

Your Nutrition Solution Tidbit: Infection from *H. pylori* is more common than you might think. More than a billion people around the world are affected by this bacterium, with an estimated 50 percent of the U.S. population over the age of 60 years. Not everyone affected by *H. pylori* will develop peptic ulcer disease, but as of this writing it is estimated that 20 percent of all ulcers are associated with *H. pylori*. Eliminating the *H. pylori* bacteria with antibiotics has shown to heal the ulcers and help prevent their reoccurrence.

Symptoms of peptic ulcers, and the severity of those symptoms, can vary widely from one person to the next. The following are the most common signs and symptoms:

- Burning pain in the middle or upper stomach, usually between meals and at night.

- Change in appetite.

- Nausea and/or vomiting.

- Heartburn.
- Bloating.

Severe symptoms can include dark or black stools due to bleeding; unexplained weight loss; vomiting blood; and severe pain in the middle and upper abdomen. Although acute ulcers often heal on their own, you should never ignore the symptoms and warning signs. Ulcers can sometimes become chronic and severe, and if not properly treated, can lead to serious health issues such as internal bleeding, scar tissue, and infection.

Your doctor may diagnose your ulcer simply by speaking with you about your symptoms, and may treat you by prescribing an acid-blocking medication such as those used for heartburn. He or she may also suggest dietary and other lifestyle changes. If your symptoms seem more severe or your doctor is unsure of the diagnosis, he or she may confirm the diagnosis by testing for H. pylori, performing an endoscopy (an exam of your upper digestive system), and/or scheduling an upper GI series or barium swallow exam.

If it turns out that are infected with H. pylori, you will most likely be prescribed an antibiotic. Full-blown ulcers are usually treated with medication (to reduce stomach acid) and surgery. Medications commonly used include H2 blockers (histamine type 2 antagonists) such as cimetidine (Tagamet), famotidine (Pepcid), nizatidine (Axid), and ranitidine (Zantac); or PPI's (proton pump inhibitors) such as omeprazole (Prilosec), lansoprazole (Prevacid), rabeprazole (AcipHex), pantoprazole (Protonix), esomeprazole (Nexium), and dexlansorprazole (Dexilant). Another type of PPI consists of a combination of omeprazole and sodium bicarbonate (Zegerid). Doctors normally recommend the same type of diet for ulcers and *H. pylori* as they do for acid reflux, advising patients to avoid spicy, fatty, and acidic foods, even though *H. pylori* does not cause acid reflux.

Diverticular disease

The umbrella term "diverticular disease" includes both *diverticulosis* and *diverticulitis*. Diverticulosis is the condition of having *diverticula*, small pouches or sacs that form in the wall of the large intestine that have abnormally bulged outward through weak spots. Diverticulitis occurs when diverticula become inflamed or infected. According to the National Institutes of Health (NIH), as many as one in 10 Americans over the age of 40 and about half of all people over 60 have diverticulosis.

Diverticulosis is not usually associated with symptoms unless diverticulitis occurs. In fact, many people never even know they have diverticulosis until they have a diverticulitis flare-up. The NIH states that only about 10 to 25 percent of people who have diverticulosis will actually develop the complications and symptoms of diverticulitis. The majority of people who develop diverticulitis do not end up with serious or long-term complications, but they can experience some unpleasant symptoms that can come on quite suddenly, including abdominal pain (mainly in the lower left side), chills, fever, nausea, and vomiting. More serious symptoms include bleeding, infections, fistulas, and blockages in the intestinal tract.

Experts believe that a low-fiber diet over many years may also play a role in the development of diverticular disease. A high-fiber diet along with plenty of fluid and regular exercise to help keep bowels regulated may help prevent the development of diverticular disease and help reduce the occurrence of diverticulitis in individuals with diverticulosis.

> **Your Nutrition Solution Tidbit:** Whether you've been diagnosed with diverticular disease or not, the American Dietetic Association recommends that all adults consume 20 to 35 grams of fiber each day. I discuss the topic of fiber in Chapter 2.

If your doctor suspects a problem, she can test for diverticula in a few ways, including a blood test, stool sample, rectal exam, and/or an imaging test such as a CT scan, x-ray, abdominal ultrasound, or barium enema. Because most people with diverticulosis never experience symptoms, it is often discovered through a test such as an endoscopy that is being run for another problem.

Because many people don't even realize they have diverticulosis until diverticulitis rears its ugly head, they are not able to treat it until symptoms occur. If diverticulosis is discovered, it is treated primarily with a high-fiber diet to prevent diverticulitis from developing. If diverticulitis does develop, a mild case is treated with antibiotics to knock out the infection along with a doctor-supervised liquid diet and/or low-fiber diet for a short time to help rest and heal the colon. If severe diverticulitis occurs, an individual may need to be hospitalized.

Your Nutrition Solution Tidbit: In the past, people with diverticular disease were told to avoid eating nuts, seeds, corn, and popcorn because it was believed that these food would increase the risk of developing diverticulitis, by getting caught in the diverticula, or outpouches, of the intestines. However a large 2008 study in the *Journal of American Medical Association* concluded that consumption of these foods does *not* increase the complications of diverticulosis, including diverticulitis, and that it is not necessary to eliminate these foods. (See: Strate, L. L., et al. "Nut, Corn, and Popcorn Consumption and the Incidence of Diverticular Disease." *JAMA: The Journal of the American Medical Association*, 300.8 (2008): 907–14.) In fact, eating a diet rich in fiber—including these foods—can help reduce your risk for diverticulitis. Just make sure to chew these and all the foods you eat well. Keep in mind that people differ in terms of the amounts and types of foods they can tolerate. Decisions about individual diets should be based on what works best for you, and made in conjunction with a healthcare professional.

Chronic constipation

We have all dealt with occasional constipation, but chronic constipation is no laughing matter. It is one of the chief digestive complaints among Americans. It can make you feel miserable and can lead to multiple doctor visits and inflated medication costs, both over-the-counter and prescription. Chronic constipation is defined as having a bowel movement fewer than three times per week for several consecutive months. It can also be defined as straining or having difficulty passing stools on a regular basis. This serious issue affects 15 to 20 percent of American adults.

Normally, after we eat, the food moves through the digestive tract as the intestines absorb water and nutrients from the food. As the process proceeds, the stool is formed, and the large intestine eliminates the stool from the body. Constipation occurs when the stool moves too slowly through the digestive tract, which causes it to become hard and dry and difficult to pass. Chronic constipation can be caused by:

- Blockages in the colon or rectum.
- Issues with nerves around the colon and rectum that can be the result of certain health conditions, such as stroke, Parkinson's disease, dementia, and multiple sclerosis.
- Problems with the muscles that are needed for proper elimination.
- Conditions that affect the hormones that help balance fluids in the body, such as diabetes, pregnancy, or hypothyroidism.
- Dehydration.
- Some medical issues such as irritable bowel syndrome (IBS), hypothyroidism, celiac disease, and diabetes.

Some people may be at a higher risk for chronic constipation, such as older adults, people who consistently consume a low-fiber diet, and people who get little to no physical activity. Even taking certain medications can increase your risk for chronic constipation. Culprits include sedatives, iron supplements, diuretics, antidepressants, calcium supplements, acetaminophen, aspirin, and medications that are meant to lower blood pressure.

Chronic constipation can be debilitating. It can leave you feeling bloated, crampy, headache-y, and irritable. Decreased frequency of bowel movements, hard stools, excessive straining, and sensation of a blockage can all be symptoms of chronic constipation. If you deal with any of these on a regular basis, or if experiencing constipation is something new for you, contact your doctor. Chronic constipation can be an early sign of more serious GI problems including colon cancer, inflammatory bowel disease (IBD), bacterial or viral infection, or an obstruction.

To properly diagnose you, your doctor will take a full medical history, perform a physical exam, and may order several screening tests such as a blood test, x-ray, colonic transit study, and sigmoidoscopy and/or colonoscopy to help identify the cause of your constipation. Knowing whether the cause of constipation is another health issue is important, because treating the underlying problem will most likely relieve the chronic constipation, as well.

If chronic constipation is not secondary to another health issue, relieving the chronic constipation will involve a multidisciplinary approach that includes diet, lifestyle changes, and possibly medication. An increase in dietary fiber such as that found in whole grains, ground flaxseed, beans, fruits, and vegetables, as well as increased fluid intake and physical activity, should be recommended. You might want to speak with your doctor about a magnesium supplement. Magnesium helps to relax the muscles in the intestines to provide a smoother rhythm and also helps to absorb water to soften the stool, both of which can help ease constipation. You may be referred to a gastroenterologist and a registered dietitian nutritionist (RDN), both of whom can help you manage your problem long term and improve your quality of life.

Your Nutrition Solution Tidbit: If you deal with chronic constipation don't take matters into your own hands by taking laxatives on a regular basis. Laxatives contain chemicals that will help to temporarily relieve constipation. However, when they are misused and/or overused, they can wreak havoc and actually cause chronic constipation. If your doctor has prescribed a laxative, take them only as prescribed and speak with your doctor about the length of time it is safe to use them.

Irritable bowel syndrome (IBS)

Irritable bowel syndrome (IBS) is a functional gastrointestinal (GI) disorder, which means that the symptoms are caused by changes in how the GI tract functions. IBS affects the large intestine, interfering primarily with the normal functioning of the colon. It is a chronic condition that needs to be managed long term. The symptoms of IBS may be worse or better on any given day, but the syndrome does not damage the GI tract and does not increase your risk of developing other, more serious health conditions. In fact, IBS is not classified as a disease but as a syndrome: a group of symptoms that occur together.

Experts are not quite sure what causes IBS, but they believe that certain factors may play a major role in its development. During the digestive process, the muscles that line the walls of the intestines alternately contract and relax as food moves from the stomach, through the intestinal tract, and into the rectum. In IBS, these contractions can be stronger and longer, or, just the opposite, weaker and shorter. Both ends of the spectrum cause symptoms. Dysfunctional brain-gut signals, or the signals between the brain and the nerves of the small and large intestines that control how the intestines work, can cause IBS symptoms. Another cause of IBS can be SIBO, or small intestinal bacterial overgrowth, which we will discuss in the next section. People with IBS can be more sensitive to certain triggers that bring on symptoms, but again, it will differ from person to person. These triggers or stimuli can include certain food sensitivities, large meals, stress, anxiety, depression, caffeine, hormonal changes, medications, alcohol, and certain illnesses.

Your Nutrition Solution Tidbit: IBS affects as many as three to 20 percent of all adults, with only about five to seven percent being properly diagnosed, as many people do not seek medical attention. This condition affects twice as many women as men and is usually found in people younger than 45 years of age.

The most common and frequent symptoms of IBS include abdominal pain or discomfort along with cramping, bloating, gas, mucus in the stool, diarrhea, and constipation. IBS is usually classified according to its symptoms. People either have IBS with diarrhea, with constipation, or a mix of the two. There will be times when symptoms are worse and times when it seems the IBS has completely disappeared. If you experience any of these symptoms and they become chronic or interfere with normal activities, you should see your doctor to be properly diagnosed and to rule out any other health-related issues.

To diagnose IBS your doctor will complete a thorough medical history along with a physical exam. The specific criteria for diagnosis of IBS are as follows: symptoms must have started at least six months prior; and symptoms must have occurred at least three times or more per month for the previous consecutive three months. Most of the time, your doctor can diagnose IBS by your symptoms alone. Your doctor may perform a screening blood test to check for other issues. Additional tests may be needed based on the results of the blood test and on the presence of any symptoms not common to IBS, such as weight loss, rectal bleeding, anemia, fever, and a family history of colon cancer, celiac disease, and/or inflammatory bowel disease (IBD). IBS is essentially diagnosed by ruling out other conditions. When the symptoms indicate IBS and lack any other medical explanation, IBS is usually the diagnosis.

There is no cure for IBS, but there are treatments available that can help relieve symptoms and manage the condition long term. Treatment usually involves a combination of therapies, including dietary changes, medication, supplements such as probiotics, regular exercise, and stress management. Dietary changes include avoiding foods you are personally sensitive to as well as foods that are high in fat, alcohol, caffeine, dairy (for some people), gas-causing foods, spicy foods, and beverages with large amounts of artificial sweeteners. For those whose chief symptom is constipation, dietary soluble fiber is usually increased. An important dietary approach to IBS is called the FODMAPs elimination diet. FODMAPs is an acronym for fermentable, oligo-, di- and mono-saccharides, and polyols. FODMAPs are a group of fermentable short-chain carbohydrates that are believed to cause symptoms such as gas, bloating, and watery diarrhea for some IBS suffers. We will talk more about food sensitivities and FODMAPs in Chapter 2. The most effective treatment for IBS comes from working with your doctor and a registered dietitian nutritionist (RDN) to find the individual plan that works best for you.

Gallstones

The gallbladder houses bile, an important digestive fluid that is produced by the liver, and releases it when it is needed into the small intestine. This small, pear-shaped organ is located right underneath the liver. An imbalance among the substances that make up bile can cause gallstones. If bile contains too much cholesterol, too much bilirubin, or not enough bile salts, gallstones can form. These gallstones can range in size from very tiny to the size of a golf ball; you can develop just one or many at the same time. Researchers are not quite sure why these types of imbalances in bile occur, but they do know that gallstones can form if the gallbladder does not empty completely or often enough. There are two types of gallstones: cholesterol stones and pigment stones. In Americans, gallstones are usually cholesterol stones.

Experts believe that the risk for gallstones can increase due to:

- Genetics or family history.

- Obesity.

- An increase in estrogen levels (such as occurs during pregnancy).

- Being female.

- Rapid weight loss.

- Being over the age of 40.

- Having a Native American or Mexican Americans ethnic background.

- Having diabetes, insulin resistance, or metabolic syndrome. (Metabolic syndrome is an umbrella term for a group of medical conditions that have been linked to being overweight or obese, and which can put people at risk for heart disease and type 2 diabetes.)

- Certain intestinal diseases such as Crohn's disease.

- High triglyceride levels.

- Cholesterol-lowering drugs.

- Research suggests that diets high in caloric content as well as refined grains along with low fiber increases the risk for gallstones.

Less common pigment stones tend to develop in those with cirrhosis of the liver, infection of the bile ducts, or severe anemia such as sickle cell anemia.

Gallstones don't always warn you with symptoms. In this case they are called "silent stones" and do not interfere with the functioning of the gallbladder. If a gallstone lodges in and blocks a bile duct, however, it can cause a gallbladder attack, which can include the following symptoms:

- A sudden onset of rapidly intensifying pain in the upper right portion of the abdomen and/or in the center of the abdomen, just below your breastbone.
- Back pain between the shoulder blades.
- Pain in your right shoulder.
- Nausea and vomiting.
- Other gastrointestinal symptoms such as bloating, indigestion, heartburn, and gas.

Gallbladder attacks can last from several minutes to several hours and often follow a heavy meal. The gallstone attack will subside once the gallstone moves and is no longer blocking the bile duct. If the duct remains blocked for more than a few hours, complications can occur. These might include inflammation of the gallbladder and severe damage to or infection of the gallbladder, bile ducts, and liver. If a gallbladder attack lasts more than a few hours, is intensely painful, includes fever and chills, and/or yellowing of the skin or whites of the eyes, seek medical attention immediately. The symptoms of gallstones can mimic those of other conditions such as appendicitis, ulcers, pancreatitis, and acid reflux, so make sure you see your doctor for a proper diagnosis.

Because many gallstones are "silent," they aren't usually found until tests are done for another health issue.

However, if your doctor suspects gallstones, there are several tests that may be performed to confirm the diagnosis, including:

- Blood test.

- Ultrasound.

- CAT scan (CT).

- Magnetic resonance imaging (MRI).

- Cholangiopancreatography (MRCP): specifically looks at the liver and gallbladder.

- Cholescintigraphy (HIDA SCAN): tests whether the gallbladder is contracting properly. A radioactive material is used in order to observe the movements of the gallbladder.

- Endoscopic ultrasound: uses a combination of ultrasound and endoscopy to look for gallstones

- Endoscopic retrograde cholangiopancreatography (ERCP): an endoscopy of the small intestines performed with a dye to allow bile ducts to be seen. During this procedure the doctor can often remove gallstones that have moved into and blocked the ducts.

Gallstones that don't cause symptoms or discomfort usually don't need treatment. However, if a person experiences a gallbladder attack and/or other symptoms, treatment will be necessary. At this point you will be referred to a gastroenterologist, a doctor that specializes in digestive disorders, for care and treatment. Once a person has a gallbladder attack, more are likely to follow. The usual treatment at this point is to undergo surgery (called a *cholecystectomy*) to remove the gallbladder. This type of surgery is fairly common and in fact is one of the most common surgeries performed on adults in the United States. Most of these surgeries are now done with laparoscopic techniques on an outpatient basis. Luckily the gallbladder is not an essential organ, so we can live without it. Once it is removed, the bile flows directly into the duodenum instead of being stored in the gallbladder.

If the patient cannot have surgery, other non-surgical options can be used to try to dissolve the cholesterol of the gallstones, although it can take years for them to fully dissolve, and they will most likely return years down the road. A doctor may also try ERCP, mentioned previously, to remove the stones.

To maintain a healthy gut and help prevent gallstones, maintain a healthy weight. If you are overweight or obese, make sure you lose weight in a slow and healthy manner that includes exercise (if allowed by your doctor). Consume a diet low in refined and processed foods and high in fiber. Don't skip meals, and avoid fasting of any type unless it is doctor supervised.

Your Nutrition Solution Tidbit: Other well-known gut issues include acid reflux and inflammatory bowel disease (which includes Crohn's disease and colitis), and are huge topics in and of themselves. For more information on these issues, check out two of my other books: *Your Nutrition Solution to Acid Reflux* (New Page Books, 2014), and *Tell Me What to Eat If I Have Inflammatory Bowel Disease* (New Page Books, 2011).

Is Leaky Gut Syndrome a Real Problem?

Leaky gut syndrome (or *increased intestinal permeability*) sounds like it must be just a digestive issue. However, many healthcare experts believe that this syndrome can be the cause of a host of health issues, including food allergies/sensitivities, low energy levels, joint pain, thyroid disease, skin conditions, autoimmune conditions, IBS, IBD, asthma, a slow metabolism, and the list goes on. Proponents of leaky gut syndrome believe that the filter system of the digestive tract or gut gets damaged, so things that normally can't pass through, such as undigested food particles, bacterial toxins, and germs, now can. These substances then pass through the "leaky" gut wall and into the bloodstream and trigger the immune system, causing chronic inflammation throughout the body and all types of health issues. Still other healthcare experts believe that this theory is just that: a theory that is still scientifically unproven.

Experts who believe that leaky gut syndrome is a genuine malady, believe it can be caused by poor diet, chronic stress, toxin overload, and bacterial imbalance (an imbalance between beneficial, or "good," and harmful, or "bad," gut bacteria). They recommend avoiding foods and beverages that contain gluten, GMO (genetically modified organisms) foods, cow's milk, and sugar to prevent and/or heal the health issues that a leaky gut supposedly causes.

As of this writing, the best answer to this question is that leaky gut syndrome is still greatly misunderstood, and much more research needs to be conducted before we can answer the question of whether it is genuine and the possible cause of so many health issues.

Your Nutrition Solution Tidbit: Genetically modified organisms (GMOs) were introduced into the American food supply in the mid 1990's. GMO foods are created through a laboratory process to artificially alter and/or introduce new traits or characteristics into the DNA of an organism. GMOs are produced for example to enhance the growth or nutritional content of a food crop. The majority of genetically modified (GM) food crops being used in the food market today include soybean, corn, cotton (oil), canola (oil), and beet sugar. These GM plants are typically used to make ingredients that are than used in other food products, generally processed foods, of all kinds. Although the FDA regulates and deems these GM foods safe there is much controversy surrounding them and our digestive system. Many experts, such as The Institute for Responsible Technology, believe that GMO foods are leading to impaired digestion and are the reason for the increase in gluten-sensitivity, leaky gut syndrome, and other prevalent gut issues. (Source: Smith, Jeffery M. "Are Genetically Modified Foods a Gut-Wrenching Combination?" Institute for Responsible Technology, n.d. Webpage accessed December 5, 2014.)

What Are the Causes of an Unhealthy Gut?

As you have learned, an unhealthy gut can cause more than just digestive symptoms such as gas, bloating, diarrhea, and other discomforts. Much of our immune system is located in our gut, so an unhealthy gut can mean an unhealthy you in many other ways that are not directly gut related. So what causes an unhealthy gut? It is pretty clear that lifestyle has something to do with it. In general, an unhealthy diet that is low in fiber and high in refined carbohydrates, sugar, and processed foods, and lacking in whole foods that provide essential nutrients for good health and healthy gut flora (foods such as fruits, vegetables, and whole grains), can definitely contribute to an unhealthy gut. Chronic stress, alcohol intake, smoking, infections, over-use of certain medications, including anti-inflammatories and antibiotics, a sedentary lifestyle, and obesity can be other root causes.

Another condition that you may not have heard of, called small intestinal bacterial overgrowth (SIBO), can also result in an unhealthy gut. Although the entire GI tract contains bacteria, the small intestine is one of the cleaner parts of the digestive tract, with the large intestine and colon containing the highest number. Bacteria found in the small intestine consist of different strains than those found in the large intestine. Small intestinal bacterial overgrowth (SIBO) occurs when the number of bacteria found in the small intestine increases and/or becomes imbalanced with the "bad" bacteria—some of which are the same strains found in the large intestine—thus out-numbering the "good" bacteria.

After food reaches the stomach and is prepared for digestion, it is pushed through the three discrete parts of the small intestine: the duodenum, the jejunum, and the ileum. Then it is moved into the large intestine and colon. The small intestine is where most nutrients are absorbed into the body. The muscular action that pushes the food through its journey (called *peristalsis*) sweeps bacteria out of the small intestines and thus helps limit the number of bacteria there. When something interferes with the normal process of how the food travels through the small intestine and allows bacteria to stick around and multi-ply, this can result in SIBO. Interference with the normal muscular activity can also allow bacteria from the colon to back up into the small intestines.

Some of conditions that can cause issues in the small intestines and allow SIBO to develop include neurological or muscular diseases; diabetes; scleroderma; obstruction of the small intestines, such as from scarring from pre-vious surgeries or Crohn's disease; and diverticuli (small pouches in the small intestines that allow bacteria to get stuck and multiply). SIBO is essentially a chronic infec-tion of the small intestine with the result being excessive fermentation of dietary carbohydrates that can cause vari-ous GI symptoms, including:

- Excessive flatulence/gas.
- Abdominal bloating/distention.
- Diarrhea with painful cramping.

- Constipation.

- Abdominal pain.

If the overgrowth of bacteria is severe and prolonged, the bacteria can interfere with the normal process of digestion and absorption of food, which can result in vitamin and mineral deficiencies as well as weight loss. If fat malabsorption occurs, this can lead to deficiencies of vitamin A, D, and E. Vitamin B12 deficiency is also common in SIBO. Some people with SIBO also complain of non-GI symptoms such as body aches and fatigue. Symptoms of SIBO can become chronic and come and go over periods of months or even years before they are properly diagnosed. A diagnosis of IBS can be a big red flag to probable SIBO. In fact, SIBO may be the underlying cause of many cases of IBS as well as chronic relapses of Crohn's disease, and the reason why some celiac patients don't respond as they should to a gluten-free diet. In addition, food intolerances; chronic illnesses such as fibromyalgia, chronic fatigue syndrome, autoimmune diseases, diabetes, and celiac disease; long-term use of antibiotics; and diverticulosis can all be a warning signs that SIBO may be present.

Diagnosing SIBO is not an easy task. To confirm a diagnosis, blood tests, a hydrogen breath test (which measures hydrogen and methane gas production), cultures of intestinal fluid, a stool sample test, and/or biopsies of tissue from the small intestine may be used. SIBO is frequently treated and managed with antibiotics and probiotics, or a combination of both. In addition, refined carbohydrates and sugar should be reduced or eliminated from the diet. Avoiding snacking in between meals helps give the intestines time for cleansing. Avoiding high-FODMAP foods can also be helpful and something we will discuss in Chapter 2. For some patients, oral supplements may be needed for vitamin deficiencies. Once SIBO is treated a close eye still needs to be kept, as relapses are fairly common. Relapses really depend on how well the underlying illness, the probable cause of the SIBO, is managed.

How Are Gut Issues Treated?

There are many types of gut and digestive issues that can occur, and depending on the condition at hand, treatment will vary. However, there are steps that everyone can take to create a healthier gut and lower the risk for gut-related disorders. Focusing on diet, stress management, regular exercise, and a healthy weight are certainly all keys to treating these conditions and possibly helping to prevent them. Supplements, including probiotics and prebiotics, are becoming more mainstream as a way of both treating and managing symptoms of digestive disorders as well as a means of prevention.

Can a Detoxifying Diet Help My Gut?

The idea of following a detox or "gut-cleansing" diet can sound appealing when it promises to rid your body of dangerous toxins from your gut. Detox diets are controversial at best. On one hand, we already have a built-in detox system in our body. The liver takes care of potential "toxins" by rendering them harmless, and your intestines create bacteria that "detoxify" waste. The human body comes complete with a complex detoxification system that, when cared for properly, should do the job it was meant to do. There is no scientific evidence that proves that detox diets work any better at ridding your body of dangerous toxins than your own gut, immune system, and organs already do. That said, some experts question whether everyone's natural detoxification system is up to par and always working at peak performance.

There are countless numbers of detox diets that you can find anywhere from the local drug store to online. Many are extremely restrictive. Fasting detox diets and "gut-cleansing" regimens can put you at risk for electrolyte imbalance and dehydration. Worse yet, they can do the opposite of what you are looking for and disrupt the balance of bacteria in your gut and bowels. If you are going to try a detox diet, my best advice is to avoid ones that seem dramatic, unrealistic, and/or extreme and that last for more than just a day or two. Follow guidelines that seem reasonable and safe and that promote a healthy lifestyle. Don't set yourself up for a let-down by having unrealistic expectations of what the diet will do.

A better way to detox is to make permanent lifestyle changes you can stick with. Such changes include eating a healthy and well-balanced diet, maintaining a healthy weight, fitting in regular exercise, and drinking plenty of water. All of these changes will be better at getting the results you are looking for, *and* they will last a lifetime. If you plan on trying a detox diet anyway, always consult with your doctor first.

chapter 2

the nutrition connection and beyond

If you are going to be successful at making dietary changes that benefit your gut health, the first step is to understand the strong nutrition connection that exists between the food and beverages you consume and your digestive system. Nutrition plays a crucial role in the functioning and health of the gut, as well as in managing symptoms, should they occur. This chapter will discuss the role that certain carbohydrates (sugars and refined grains) and fiber play in regulating the gut and keeping it humming at peak performance. We will also discuss foods that can cause gas, the role that food intolerances and sensitivities can play in digestive issues, some supplements and nutrients that can help support gut health, and, finally, the FODMAPs diet approach and why it might be right for you.

Our Relationship With Carbohydrates

For a lot of people, their relationship with carbohydrates is a tight and loving bond. For others, "carb" is a four-letter word. Most of us are drawn to comfort foods, which usually include sweets such as ice cream, cake, candy, and cookies, and more savory treats such as bread, chips, and French fries. What do all these foods have in common? They are all chock full of carbohydrates. Carbohydrates, or "carbs," along with proteins and fats, are the main sources of calories in our diets. Carbs are essential in that they provide fuel for our body in the form of glucose. They are found mainly in fruits, vegetables (especially starchy vegetables), dairy products, bread, cereal, rice, pasta, and anything containing sugar. Unlike proteins and fats, carbs are broken down directly into sugar very early in the digestive process. When it comes to carbohydrates and your gut, the problem lies in two specific types of carbohydrates: sugar and refined starches. We don't worry as much about the beneficial carbs such as whole grains and the fiber they contain.

There are three main types of carbohydrates in food:

1. **Sugars** (also called *simple carbohydrates* or *simple sugars*) contain either one unit of sugar (these are

called *monosaccharides*) or two (these are called *disaccharides*). These simple sugars are broken down quickly and cause a quick rise in blood sugar. They come in two main categories: naturally occurring sugars, such as the sugar found in fruits and dairy products; and added sugars, such as those added during processing.

2. **Starches** (also called *complex carbohydrates*) are single sugars that are bonded together. They are broken down into simple carbohydrates or sugars during digestion, and are processed more slowly than simple sugars are in the body. This results in a more gradual rise in blood sugar. Complex carbohydrates can be found in starchy vegetables (peas, corn, and potatoes); dried beans and lentils; and grains (both refined and whole) such as wheat, oats, and barley.

3. **Fiber,** also considered a carbohydrate, comes strictly from plant foods and is the indigestible part of these foods. Good sources of fiber include whole grains, fruits, vegetables, beans, and nuts.

Both complex carbohydrates and fiber are needed by the gut to help produce "friendly" or "good" bacteria. The Dietary Guidelines for Americans recommends that carbohydrates comprise 45 to 65 percent of total daily calories. So, for example, if you consume 2,000 calories per day, 900 to 1,300 of those calories should come from carbohydrates; that works out to be about 225 to 325 grams. Most Americans consume plenty of carbohydrates; the problem is that they consume more of the wrong type, the refined starches and sugar, and less of the right kind, whole grains and fiber.

> **Your Nutrition Solution Tidbit:** A small study in applied and environmental microbiology raised concerns about the impact of low-carbohydrate diets on gut health. The researchers found that prolonged use of a low-carb diet had an adverse effect on the production of specific "friendly" bacteria that are needed to produce a substance called *butyrate*, which is important for gut health and for helping to prevent colon cancer. (Source: Duncan, Sylvia H., Alvaro Belenguer, et al. "Reduced Dietary Intake of Carbohydrates by Obese Subjects Results in Decreased Concentrations of Butyrate and Butyrate-Producing Bacteria in Feces." *Applied and Environmental Microbiology.* 73.4 (2007): 1073–78. American Society for Microbiology. Webpage accessed January 1, 2015.) So before you hit that low-carb diet to lose weight, you might want to think again!

Grains: Understanding the difference

Grains come in two different forms, and the two couldn't be more different as far as gut health is concerned. Refined grains have been milled (or refined), which is a process that removes the bran and germ from the grain, leaving only the endosperm. This also removes essential nutrients and fiber. Foods with refined grains include white flour, white rice, white bread, sugary cereals, and white pasta, just to name a few. Many refined grains are enriched, meaning some of the nutrients that were lost after the refining process are added back in. However, fiber is not one of them, so refined grains have a much lower fiber content than their whole counterparts. Most importantly for the topic of this book, refined grains can have a negative impact on our gut health.

Whole grains include the entire grain kernel: bran, germ, and endosperm. These grains are high in complex carbohydrates and rich in fiber. In addition, they contain large amounts of B vitamins and vitamin E. Whole grains are a good source of iron, zinc, selenium, and magnesium.

Your Nutrition Solution Tidbit: When choosing whole-grain foods, look for the word "whole" on the label or in the ingredient list so you know it is truly a whole grain. For example, if the label on a loaf of bread states that it is "wheat" bread, it is not made entirely of whole grains but probably a combination of whole-wheat and refined flours. Don't be fooled by the brown color of these breads: caramel coloring is commonly used to make refined products look brown hence healthier. On the other hand, if a loaf of bread states "whole wheat," then it is made with 100-percent whole wheat flour. The Food and Drug Administration (FDA) defines whole-grain foods as those foods containing

51 percent or more whole-grain ingredients by weight. Check out *http://wholegrainscouncil. org* for more info on whole grains.

The choice between whole and refined grains is an easy one. For better overall health, a healthier gut, and help in managing gut issues you may already have, whole grains are your best choice. Try to increase your intake of whole grains as you reduce the amount of refined grains you consume.

Not sure about sugar?

Sugar is a refined carbohydrate. As I mentioned previously, it can be added to foods or beverages in processing, or it can be a natural part of foods such as fruit (fructose) or milk and milk products (lactose). There are many different names for added sugars, including table sugar, honey, cane sugar, molasses, syrup, high-fructose corn syrup, powdered sugar, raw sugar, beet sugar, invert sugar, and brown sugar. Sometimes you will find sugar listed by its chemical name such as dextrose, sucrose, glucose, lactose, maltose, or fructose. You can recognize other chemical names for sugar as they all end in "-ose."

Sugar may be a delight to your taste buds, but your gut can do without it. Sugar encourages bad gut bacteria to reproduce, flourish, and overwhelm your gut. Sugar is also the number-one source of calories in the typical American diet, provides no nutritional value, and is one of the biggest causes of overweight/obesity in the American population. An unhealthy gut and unwanted weight are just two of the problems that can arise from the overconsumption of sugar and sugary foods. In general, people who eat large amounts of added sugar tend to have diets that are low in calcium, vitamin A, iron, zinc, and dietary fiber. A 2010 study in the *Journal of the American Medical Association* found that people who ate the most added sugar had the lowest HDL (good cholesterol) and the highest blood triglyceride levels (blood fats), both of which are major risk factors for heart disease. (Source: Welsh, J.A., A. Sharma, et al. "Caloric Sweetener Consumption and Dyslipidemia among U.S. Adults." *Journal of the American Medical Association*, 303.15 (2010): 1490–497. National Center for Biotechnology Information. U.S. National Library of Medicine/PubMed.gov.)

Foods that contain natural sugars, such as fruits, dairy products, and some vegetables, are quite a different story. These foods contain naturally occurring sugars but also contain essential nutrients that are vital for good health and a healthy gut, such as fiber, vitamins, minerals, antioxidants, and phytonutrients. These foods, even though they contain simple sugars, are not processed or refined and thus are not a detriment to your gut. So there is no excuse to not eat your fruit and veggies and drink your milk!

Fiber facts

You learned in Chapter 1 that fiber is a significant way to a healthier gut and better overall health in general. But do you really know what fiber is and where to get it? Dietary fiber is a substance found only in plants, more specifically, in the plant cell walls that provide plants with their shape and structure. Although the body cannot digest or absorb fiber, it provides some amazing health benefits as it travels through the digestive tract. Fiber is a type of complex carbohydrate, but because it doesn't provide nutritional value, it is not considered a nutrient per se. However, you can still find it listed on food nutrient labels to help you identify foods rich in fiber.

Not all dietary fiber is created equal. All fiber falls into one of two categories: *soluble* fiber and *insoluble* fiber. They differ in their ability to dissolve in water as well as their effect on the body. They are both equally important to our health, however. The key is to eat a variety of fiber-rich foods each day in order to get enough of both types. Many foods contain both types of fiber, although many contain more of one type of fiber over the other.

Soluble fiber is just that: soluble in water. It both soothes and regulates the digestive tract. By absorbing water and forming a gel-like consistency, it helps slow down digestion and the movement of food through the intestines. For those who suffer from chronic diarrhea and IBS, soluble fiber can be very beneficial. Soluble fiber produces softer stools, which can help to relieve chronic constipation, as well. This type of fiber tends not to cause irritation and inflammation, so it can help to relieve abdominal cramping. Soluble fiber also provides the major health benefit of lowering LDL, or "bad" blood cholesterol level, which in turn can help reduce your risk for heart disease. Finally, soluble fiber also slows down the rate at which glucose is absorbed by the body. This can help to control blood sugar levels in people with diabetes and other blood sugar issues. Foods that contain higher amounts of soluble fiber include:

- Dried beans and peas.
- Fruits such as apricots, bananas, apples, pears, citrus fruits, peaches, prunes, plums, mangoes, and grapes (does not include the peel).
- Vegetables such as Brussel's sprouts, beets, peeled potatoes, carrots, squash, pumpkin, cauliflower, and broccoli.
- Oats, bran, and barley
- Brown rice.
- Avocados.
- Psyllium seeds.

Insoluble fiber is the fiber that adds bulk to food, which helps it move along the intestinal tract helping to avoid constipation, hemorrhoids, and promote regularity, which is critical in maintaining a healthy gut. Unlike soluble fiber, insoluble fiber does not dissolve in water; rather, it actually draws water *into* the GI tract, thus allowing the digestive tract to keep things in motion. Insoluble fibers usually reside on the outside of foods and the soluble part resides on the inside for most foods. For example the skin of an apple contains insoluble fiber and the inside contains soluble fibers.

Foods that include high amounts of insoluble fiber include:

- Whole-grain breads, pastas, and cereals.
- Whole-grain flours.
- Brown rice and wild rice.
- Wheat bran.

- Nuts and seeds.

- Popcorn.

- Beans and lentils.

- Fruits such as berries, grapes, raisins, cherries, pine-apples, peaches, apples with skin, oranges, prunes, melons, and grapefruits.

- Vegetables such as spinach, kale, peas, corn, green beans, peppers, celery, onions, broccoli, cauliflower, and tomatoes.

A diet high in a both types of fiber can help gut health in so many ways. It increases stool bulk and speeds the passage of stools through the bowel, thus helping to prevent colon cancer, diverticulitis, and IBS, as well as many other GI conditions. Eating plenty of fiber can also help suppress hunger and make you feel fuller longer, which in turn can help with weight loss or maintaining a healthy weight.

A Gassy Problem

We all have it, whether we like to admit it or not. Gas, or *flatulence*, in more technical terms, is a very normal occurrence. The body produces gas in the stomach and the intestines during the normal digestive process. Air that is swallowed while eating too quickly, or while chewing gum or sucking on candy, can also produce gas. Increasing your fiber intake too quickly or eating too much at once, especially if your GI system isn't quite used to it yet, can also cause gas issues. The normal person passes gas anywhere from six to 20 times a day. If you are passing gas more often than that, it could be a warning sign of a problem in the gut. Possible causes of excess gas include celiac disease, Crohn's disease, reflux disease, IBS, lactose intolerance, fructose malabsorption, a food sensitivity, peptic ulcer disease, and ulcerative colitis. If you have excessive gas, it is a good idea to see your doctor. There could be an underlying reason; or, it could be a sign that you are not managing a previously diagnosed GI issue properly.

Sometimes gas comes from foods that we consume. Some foods and beverages tend to cause more gas than others. You already know that too many fiber-rich foods too quickly can lead to gas. If you are lactose intolerant, foods that contain dairy, such as milk, cheese, and ice cream, may cause gas issues for you. In addition, a high-fat diet can be the culprit as it tends to produce more gas in the system. The following foods tend to cause gas more often than others. This doesn't mean you need to completely avoid these foods; in fact, many of the foods listed are very healthy ones. Everyone is different, so your best bet is to figure out which foods bother you the most by trial and error. Eliminate some or all of these foods from your diet and begin to add them back in slowly, one at a time, to figure out which one is the culprit. Once you are pretty sure you know what your problem foods are, eat small amounts of those foods initially, increasing the portion size slowly until you know the amount that you can eat without the unwanted side effect. (Note that this is not an all-inclusive list; there will be foods that bother you that may not be on here.)

Foods that tend to cause gas include, but are not limited to:

- Asparagus
- Broccoli
- Brussel's sprouts
- Cabbage
- Cauliflower
- Onions
- Peppers
- Sauerkraut
- Apples
- Bananas
- Citrus fruits
- Prunes and prune juice
- Raisins
- Dried beans
- Carbonated beverages
- Eggs
- Whole grains
- Sugar alcohols such as sorbitol or xylitol

Uncovering Beneficial Dietary Gut Supplements

Sometimes we can use a little help in our pursuit of a gut-healthy diet and lifestyle, and in our efforts to manage symptoms or prevent issues from developing in the first place. As we age, we naturally lose some of those friendly bacteria that we have come to know so well; the power of our immune system diminishes, as well. This can increase our susceptibility to all types of GI disorders and health issues. Following are a few dietary supplements that are definitely worth a look.

Probiotics

Probiotics are the helpful and friendly living microorganisms—microbes, bacteria, and yeast—that are found in our gut. They are a functional and natural component of foods and supplements that may help to boost immunity and improve overall health, especially gut health. Probiotics can be found in foods such as yogurt, kefir (fermented milk), miso, tempeh, some juices, and soy beverages. Supplements come in many forms, including capsules, tablets, and powders. A number of different bacteria are used in probiotic supplements, and they all have different effects, depending on the strain. These bacteria might include *Bifidobacterium,* which you can also find in some dairy products and can help ease symptoms of IBS; and *Lactobacillus,* one of the most common probiotics that can be found in yogurt and other fermented foods. Probiotic supplements can help to replenish "good" bacteria in your gut as you age and/or after you take a round of antibiotics. They can also help to lower the number of "bad" bacteria in your gut. And they can help to balance the "good" and "bad" bacteria to keep your gut working efficiently. Although research is still ongoing, probiotics have been found to help with infectious diarrhea, effects from *H. pylori*, colitis caused by *C. diff*, ulcerative colitis, IBS, chronic constipation, diarrhea caused by antibiotics, and inflammation of the GI tract. They may also help relieve Crohn's disease and help prevent allergies, yeast infections, urinary tract infections, and some skin issues. This doesn't mean they are a cure-all for whatever ails your gut, but they can help to relieve symptoms and flare-ups and possibly prevent problems from surfacing.

To work efficiently, probiotic supplements must have enough good bacteria to allow them to grow in the gut. When choosing a probiotic supplement, always check the "best by" date, as these supplements tend to lose their potency pretty quickly. If a product does not list a "best by" date, the product probably contains minimal or no live bacteria at the time of purchase and/or consumption, and therefore will not be as effective. Supplements are usually sensitive to heat, moisture, and air and many need to be refrigerated. Each specific probiotic tends to be most effective for a certain illness or condition, so knowing which one to choose is important. Although exactly which one to take, and how often to take it, will depend on your doctor's recommendation, a probiotic supplement that includes one to 10 billion CFU's (colony forming units), once per day, is the typical dosage.

The Food and Drug Administration (FDA) regulates probiotic supplements as foods instead of as medications. Therefore, unlike drug companies, the makers of probiotic supplements do not have to prove that their products are safe and/or effective. However, in general, probiotic supplements are considered safe. Mild side effects can sometimes include upset stomach, diarrhea, gas, and/or bloating for the first few days of starting them. Ask your doctor for more information on a product and dose that is right for you.

Your Nutrition Solution Tidbit: A probiotic product called VSL#3 has been shown to be very beneficial for those with IBS.

Prebiotics

If you have heard of probiotics, chances are you have also heard of prebiotics. Prebiotics are natural, non-digestible carbohydrates that act as "food" for probiotics to flourish and do their thing. They are basically "good"-bacteria promoters. You can take prebiotics as a supplement, just like probiotics. Prebiotics have other important health benefits than just increasing intestinal flora. They can help to reduce blood triglycerides, cholesterol, and very low-density lipoproteins (VLDL), which are even worse than LDL, or "bad" cholesterol. Prebiotics can reduce the glycemic response (blood sugar response) to eating, improve water and electrolyte balance, and increase the absorption of minerals such as calcium, magnesium, iron, and zinc.

Prebiotics that promote the growth of the "good" bacteria in the gut come mostly from *oligosaccharides*. Since they do not get digested they are able to remain available in the GI tract to help promote the growth of beneficial bacteria. Two groups of oligosaccharides include *fructans* or *fructo-oligosaccharides* (FOS), which include *inulin* and *phlein*; and *glacto-oligosaccharides* (GOS). Another prebiotic is oat gum, which is rich in antioxidants as well as a kind of soluble fiber called *beta-glucan*. *Pectin* is still another prebiotic that has been shown to have powerful antioxidant effects.

Prebiotics can be found in a wide variety of foods, especially ones that are high in fiber, such as fruits, vegetables, and whole grains. Good sources include artichokes, asparagus, apples, bananas, onions, garlic, leeks, chicory, barley, quinoa, soybeans, millet, oats, berries, legumes, and whole-wheat foods.

> **Your Nutrition Solution Tidbit:** We know the great gut benefits that probiotics and prebiotics have. Combine them and they become *synbiotics*. Yogurt is an example of a synbiotic. Combine foods such as bananas on top of your yogurt for a winning combination.

As of this writing, prebiotics are being researched to determine what effects they may have on IBD, IBS, and weight control, as well as their possible use in the treatment and prevention of diarrhea and constipation. As with probiotics, different strains are more effective than others for different conditions. Current research on pre- and probiotics will continue to pave the way for their future use as a natural nutritional treatment for a wide variety of health conditions.

Digestive enzymes

Digestive enzymes occur naturally in our bodies. Working in conjunction with stomach acid, they aid in the digestion and breakdown of food into smaller, more absorbable, and more digestible components. An enzyme called *amylase* breaks down starches into sugar molecules;

protease breaks down proteins into amino acids; and *lipase* enzymes break down fat into its absorbable form. Digestive enzymes go hand-in-hand with gastric acids because it takes the acids to activate the all-important enzymes. Enzymes can be found not only in our bodies but also in some fresh foods; cooked and processed foods lack sufficient enzymes and therefore require more effort from your body. In addition, the use of acid-blocking medication for acid reflux or gastric ulcers can also lead to reduced digestive enzyme function. If your body comes up short on enzymes, for whatever reason, it can delay gastric emptying, which in turn can play a role in some gut issues. There is no concrete scientific evidence as of yet that digestive enzyme supplements are beneficial for gut health; however, they have shown promising results for some people in alleviating symptoms and improving overall digestive health. There are many digestive enzyme products on the market today. Look for products that contain all of the necessary enzymes for breaking down all of the food components, including lipase (for fat), protease (for protein), and amylase (for carbohydrates). Taking digestive enzymes before meals or at least within 30 minutes of consuming a meal is recommended.

Glutamine

Glutamine is a non-essential amino acid that is produced mainly by our muscle tissue. (Amino acids are the building blocks of protein.) It is considered non-essential because a healthy human body makes plenty, so we don't need to rely on food to get it. Glutamine is needed for rapidly dividing cells, such as the cells in the gut and the immune system. This is why if a decrease in muscle mass occurs, it can result in functional disturbances of the gut and/or immune system. In addition, during times of stress such as illness or trauma, the body has a more difficult time producing sufficient amounts of glutamine. When this happens, the amino acid becomes essential because your body cannot make enough, so a supplement may be needed. Research has shown that supplementing with glutamine can both effectively protect against and repair the damage of ulcers that are caused by H. pylori.

As a supplement, glutamine comes in the form of L-glutamine. You can find it in powder, capsule, tablet, or liquid form. Tablets and capsules generally come in 500 milligram (mg) dosages. The safe standard dose for adults 18 years and older is 500 mg, one to three times daily. Your doctor may prescribe higher doses if needed. Because this supplement can interact with certain medications, it is best to speak with your doctor first. If using a powder form, do not use in hot liquids, as heat destroys amino acids. People with kidney or liver disease or Reye's syndrome should not take glutamine. This can include elderly people who may have decreased kidney function and would need a reduced dose. You can find glutamine naturally in plant and animal proteins including beef, pork, poultry, dairy products, raw spinach, raw parsley, and cabbage.

Zinc carnosine

Zinc carnosine is a dietary supplement that consists of zinc, an essential trace mineral, and L-carnosine, an amino acid. This supplement, in conjunction with necessary diet changes, is frequently used in the treatment of gastric ulcers, especially those caused by *H. pylori*. Zinc plays a role in the synthesis of DNA (deoxyribonucleic acid) and RNA (ribonucleic acid), both of which map out our body's genetic make-up. In addition zinc has important antibacterial effects and immune-strengthening properties. L-carnosine is an amino acid that is naturally present in muscle and nerve cells and is believed to have antioxidant properties. It is the L-carnosine that seems to transport the zinc carnosine to the problem area, where it adheres to gastric mucosa and provides protective and healing effects. In addition, zinc carnosine may help to inhibit the growth of *H. pylori* and may help with other GI issues, such as symptoms from acid reflux. The most common dosage for zinc carnosine is 75 mg, twice daily.

Food Allergies, Intolerances, Sensitivities, and Your Gut

There is a fine but important line between food intolerances, food sensitivities, and food allergies. It is important to have a good understanding of what each entails and the differences among them.

Food allergies

A food allergy is the least common of the three and always triggers an immune response. An antibody called immunoglobulin E (IgE) plays a major role in the reaction by binding to the allergen and triggering the release of substances from mast cells that then cause inflammation. When the IgE binds to the mast cells, allergic reactions are initiated. This can be anything from hives to life-threatening anaphylactic shock. More common food allergy offenders include cow's milk, hen's eggs, peanuts, soy foods, wheat, fish, shellfish, and tree nuts (almonds, cashews, walnuts, pecans, pistachios, Brazil nuts, hazelnuts, and chestnuts).

Food intolerances

A food intolerance is a non-IgE allergy, non-immune digestive system response that occurs when the GI tract is unable to properly digest a particular food. Symptoms can include gas, cramps, bloating, nausea, stomach pain, vomiting, diarrhea, heartburn, headaches, and irritability. One common example of a food intolerance is lactose intolerance; another, lesser-known intolerance is fructose intolerance/malabsorption. Many factors can contribute to a food intolerance. It can be the lack of a specific enzyme, as in lactose intolerance; or it can be an intolerance to a chemical ingredient, such as added food coloring or sulfites. Food intolerances can be tough to diagnose but can usually be discovered through trial and error to determine which food is causing the problem. An elimination diet can also be helpful in pinpointing the culprit, as can a blood test and/or a skin prick test.

Lactose intolerance

Lactose intolerance occurs when your body lacks or doesn't make enough of the necessary enzyme, lactase (found in the small intestines), to break down lactose, which is the naturally occurring sugar found in milk and other dairy products. As a result, when you eat lactose-containing foods, you may experience diarrhea, bloating, and abdominal cramping. Certain health conditions, especially those dealing with the GI tract, can create a lactase deficiency later in life; for some people it just develops naturally with age.

If you suspect you are having problems digesting lactose, there are a few simple tests that can be performed to help confirm lactose intolerance. One is the hydrogen breath test; another is the stool acidity test. It is best to know for sure that lactose is causing your problem, so that you aren't avoiding dairy products needlessly. If you are lactose intolerant, you need to determine just how much lactose you can comfortably consume at one time and how many times a day your body can manage it without symptoms. Some people can tolerate lactose as long as they consume lactose-containing foods in combination with other foods. The only way to know for sure is through trial and error. Because the symptoms of lactose intolerance can mimic those of so many other GI issues, it is a good idea to see your doctor if you are experiencing symptoms.

Your Nutrition Solution Tidbit: An intolerance to lactose is not the same thing as a milk allergy. Milk allergies are quite rare and mostly affect children, who usually grow out of them by adulthood.

There are varying degrees of lactose intolerance. Some people can tolerate a little more or a little less than others. If you have a very low tolerance for lactose, you may have to avoid more than just dairy products; you may also need

to avoid products containing whey, curds, milk byprod-
ucts, dry milk solids, and non-fat dry milk powder. There
are often small amounts of lactose in breads, bread products, pastries, breakfast cereals, instant potatoes, margarine, salad dressings, cookies mixes, and many other foods.
Make sure to always read your labels if you need to avoid
lactose completely. On the other hand, some people can
tolerate small amounts of lactose, especially when it's in
yogurt that contains active cultures. So again, it is a trial-
and-error process to find out what works for you.

The biggest concern for people who are lactose intolerant is making sure they continue to get the essential
nutrients found in milk and dairy products, such as calcium and vitamin D. Non-dairy foods that contain calcium
include dark leafy greens; broccoli; canned sardines, tuna,
and salmon; calcium-fortified juices and cereals; calcium-
fortified soy products; and almonds. You can also try a
lactose-free milk that is fortified with additional nutrients.
You need vitamin D to help absorb the calcium in your
body. Most of us get vitamin D by being out in the sun for
short periods of time, but for those who are not always in
a sunny environment, this can be tough. Vitamin D can
also be found in fortified orange juice, fortified soy milk,
fatty fish such as salmon, egg yolks, and liver. If you are
not sure how to include the missing nutrients from dairy
products into your diet, speak with your doctor about
supplements and to a dietitian to look at alternate foods.

Fructose intolerance/malabsorption

Fructose malabsorption is a digestive disorder in
which the complete absorption of fructose is impaired by

deficient fructose carriers in the small intestine. The result is an increased concentration of fructose in the intestines, including the large intestine and colon, where our normal gut bacteria rapidly devour it. This results in the bacteria producing gas, which causes symptoms such as bloating/distention, cramping, gas, and sometimes diarrhea. These symptoms can closely mimic that of lactose intolerance as well as many other GI disorders. A hydrogen breath test can be done to diagnose fructose malabsorption. In addition to or in lieu of a hydrogen breath test, an elimination diet, initiated and monitored by a dietitian, can also be done to help confirm a diagnosis.

Fructose is a sugar that can be found in fruits (naturally occurring), honey, high-fructose corn syrup, corn syrup solids, fruit juice concentrate, and many processed foods. In addition you can find fructans, a form of fructose, in wheat and even some vegetables. Although all fruits contain fructose, apples, pears, honeydew melon, mangos, peaches, and watermelon contain the highest amounts. Fructose malabsorption is commonly treated with a low-fructose/fructan diet, such as the FODMAP diet approach. (I will discuss the FODMAP diet in greater depth later in this chapter.) As with lactose in lactose intolerance, everyone has a different tolerance for fructose. Doing an elimination diet and/or FODMAP diet, under the supervision of a dietitian, will help you to find your own individual tolerance level for dietary fructose.

Food sensitivities

A food sensitivity is a non-IgE allergy, immune response. Symptoms come in many forms, including acid reflux, nausea, abdominal cramps, diarrhea, and so on. With allergies and intolerances, symptoms are apparent fairly quickly after an offending food is consumed. With food sensitivities, however, someone may consume a food with no apparent symptoms and then sporadically show signs of acid reflux, headaches, nausea, abdominal cramps, and other digestive issues without being able to figure out why. This makes diagnosing food sensitivities and pinpointing specific foods and/or ingredients pretty difficult. Tools such as an oral food challenge or trial elimination diet are often used. A well-known food sensitivity is that to gluten, which includes celiac disease and non-celiac gluten sensitivity (NCGS). We will talk about both later on in this chapter.

Mediator release test (MRT)

Another way to find out whether you are suffering with food sensitivities is called a mediator release test (MRT). A MRT is a blood test that measures your immune reaction or sensitivity to a whole host of not just foods, but also additives, chemicals, and more. With the results of the MRT, your healthcare practitioner will be able to identify a list of foods and/or ingredients that you may be sensitive to and that may be the underlying cause of digestive issues. The MRT has been shown to have the highest level of accuracy of any food sensitivity blood test. This type of testing can often help to identify culprits that cannot be singled out any other way. The hub of the immune system is the gut, and when someone consumes a food that he has a reaction or a sensitivity to, the immune system sends out chemical mediators such as histamine, cytokine, and prostaglandin, all of which can produce damaging effects on body tissues and cause digestive symptoms and other major health issues. Depending on the types of mediators released, different areas of the body are affected. For example, for some people, consuming a particular food will cause migraines, for others, arthritis or maybe acid reflux. Identifying the harmful substance is the first step toward improving symptoms. Once the causative agent is identified, the next step involves following an individualized LEAP eating plan.

LEAP stands for lifestyle, eating, and performance. LEAP is an effective protocol that combines the results of the mediator release test (MRT) with the professional skills of a certified LEAP therapist (CLT). Guided by the results of the MRT test, the CLT will produce a patient-specific diet to reduce symptoms. A certified LEAP therapist—usually a dietitian—receives advanced clinical training in adverse food reactions, including food allergies, food sensitivities, and food intolerances. CLTs are trained to assist clients with the LEAP diet protocols that are based directly on the results of their MRT blood test.

You can speak with your doctor concerning LEAP therapy and MRT testing or visit *http://nowleap.com*. There is also a list of LEAP RDs and RDNs in the resource section of this book to help get you started. Many will counsel you by phone, so you don't necessarily need to reside in the same area.

Your Nutrition Solution Tidbit: Once a discovery is made and you have been diagnosed with either a food allergy, food intolerance, or food sensitivity, your doctor/allergist should refer you to a registered dietitian nutritionist for further instruction on how to handle your diet in order to eliminate the food or foods that are causing you problems while still maintaining a healthy intake.

Celiac disease

Celiac disease is an autoimmune inflammatory disorder of the small intestine that has no cure. As of this writing celiac disease is considered a food sensitivity, not an allergy, to gluten. It involves an immunological response, but not an IgE allergy response. People with celiac disease must follow a diet that is 100-percent gluten-free, as this is presently the only form of treatment. For people with celiac disease, consuming a food or beverage that contains any amount of gluten causes their body to produce specific antibodies that attack the small intestine. These antibodies destroy the *villi* (the little hairs within the lining of the small intestine) as well as digestive enzymes. Once the villi in the small intestines are destroyed, the body loses its ability to absorb nutrients needed for good health, nutrients such as carbohydrates, protein, fats, vitamins, minerals, and other essential, disease-fighting phytonutrients. Nutritional deficiencies along with the destruction of the lining of the small intestine can lead to numerous GI symptoms as well serious health conditions, both short and long term.

Because the symptoms of celiac disease mimic those of so many other digestive conditions, such as IBS and IBD, it is commonly misdiagnosed. A blood test will tell your doctor if celiac disease is a possibility, although further testing will be required in order to confirm the diagnosis. Symptoms can include many of the following:

- Reoccurring abdominal bloating and pain.
- Pale and foul-smelling stool.
- Nausea and vomiting.
- Diarrhea.
- Constipation.
- Chronic alternating diarrhea with constipation.
- Excessive flatulence.
- Bone or joint pain.
- Muscle cramps.
- Weight loss.
- Depression.
- Iron deficiency with or without unexplained anemia.
- In children, failure to thrive.

Other health conditions that can occur secondary to celiac disease include lactose intolerance, osteoporosis, tooth enamel defects, central and peripheral nervous system disease, pancreatic disease, vitamin K deficiency (associated with an increased risk for hemorrhaging), organ disorders of the gallbladder, liver and/or spleen problems, and gynecological disorders such as amenorrhea, miscarriage, and infertility. People who have celiac disease and do not adhere strictly to a gluten-free diet stand a greater chance of developing cancer in the gastrointestinal area, as well.

Once a person with celiac disease begins a gluten-free diet, the tissues of the small intestines begin to heal, and associated symptoms begin to diminish. However, just because the intestine heals doesn't mean that person can stop following a gluten-free diet. Any ingestion of gluten will start the destruction all over again, so a gluten-free diet needs to be followed closely for a lifetime.

Gluten is a protein found in wheat, rye, barley, and any derivative of these grains. A gluten-free food is completely devoid of these proteins. Foods that are naturally gluten-free include fresh fruits and vegetables, potatoes, rice, legumes, poultry, meat, and fish. Most dairy products are gluten-free and only cause a problem if you are lactose intolerant. In addition to the many naturally gluten-free fresh foods, there are many gluten-free, ready-made foods available on the market, including cereals, muffins, breads, pastas, snacks, soups, and the list goes on. Many restaurants have also joined the gluten-free train and offer special menu items and meals that are labeled as gluten-free. Gluten sneaks into foods in ways you would never think; most of the time, the word "gluten" is not even listed as an ingredient. Learning from a health professional (such as a registered dietitian nutritionist, or RDN) how to read labels properly and recognize gluten-containing ingredients is the key to success.

Your Nutrition Solution Tidbit: Celiac disease is a complex condition. If this section has piqued your curiosity and you want to know more about this disease and its treatment, check out my book *Tell Me What to Eat If I Have Celiac Disease* (Career Press, 2009) for more information.

Non-celiac gluten sensitivity (NCGS)

Some people experience food-induced reactions when consuming gluten but test negative for celiac disease and wheat allergy. Like celiac disease, NCGS involves an immunological response but no IgE allergy response. People with NCGS do not have a genetic predisposition to celiac disease, nor do they have a heightened risk of developing other autoimmune conditions, malignancies, or damage to the small intestine. There are currently no definitive diagnostic tests available for NCGS; an internal biopsy—the gold standard for diagnosing celiac disease—would have normal results because the small intestine doesn't present with damage. For people who seem to feel better on a gluten-free diet but who have tested negative for both celiac disease and a wheat allergy, the default diagnosis is usually NCGS. People with NCGS can experience many of the same symptoms as those of celiac disease, including abdominal pain, bloating, diarrhea, constipation, headaches, joint pain, chronic fatigue, depression, a "foggy" brain, and others, when they consume gluten. Similar to celiac disease, there is no "cure" for NCGS other than consuming a 100-percent gluten-free diet.

Your Nutrition Solution Tidbit: Never self-diagnose. If you have symptoms and think you may have celiac disease or gluten sensitivity, speak with your doctor before treating yourself with a gluten-free diet. Starting a gluten-free diet before having tests done can skew your test results and make diagnosis more difficult. Celiac disease can be a serious disorder, and it is essential to be accurately diagnosed as soon as possible.

The FODMAP Diet Approach

The FODMAP diet approach is used by nutrition experts to help treat some gut disorders, especially IBS. You already know that FODMAP is an acronym for fermentable, oligosaccharides, disaccharides, monosaccharides, and polyols. FODMAPs are fermentable short-chain carbohydrates (sugars and fiber) that are basically fast food for gut bacteria. When the bacteria feast on these FODMAPs, it causes GI symptoms such as gas, bloating, and watery diarrhea for some people, especially IBS suffers. These FODMAP carbohydrates include lactose, fructose, fructans (FOS), sugar alcohols, and galactans (GOS). This diet approach looks at the total amount of these types of carbohydrates that are consumed instead of looking at each type of sugar individually. In addition to being a treatment for IBS, elimination of FODMAPs may also help to alleviate symptoms of IBD (Crohn's disease and ulcerative colitis).

Oligosaccharides

Fructans are chains of fructose molecules. Fructans cannot be absorbed because the small intestine cannot break them down. This can lead to bloating, gas, and pain for some people. Wheat provides the largest amount of fructans in most people's diets. Other sources of fructans include inulin and fructo-oligosaccharide (FOS), which are commonly added to foods to increase fiber content.

Galactans, or GOS, are chains of galactose molecules. Our bodies lack the enzyme to break these sugars down into digestible components, leading to gas and other GI symptoms. Galactan-rich foods include lentils, chickpeas, beans, broccoli, cabbage, Brussel's sprouts, and soy-based products.

Disaccharides

Lactose is milk sugar, the sugar found naturally in dairy products. People who are lactose intolerant have little to none of the enzyme lactase that breaks down lactose. This means that the lactose is poorly absorbed, which causes symptoms such as abdominal bloating, pain, gas, and diarrhea. This can be quite common in celiac disease, IBS, and IBD.

Monosaccharides

Fructose is the natural sugar found in fruits. It can also be found in honey, high fructose corn syrup (HFCS), agave, and fructans. However, some fruits and fructose containing foods will be better tolerated than others.

Polyols

Polyols are also known as sugar alcohols. They are found naturally in some fruits and vegetables and are added to sugar-free products such as chewing gum, candy, and even some medications. They include sorbitol, xylitol, mannitol, erithrytol, and glycerol, just to name a few. These polyols can have a laxative effect if too many are consumed at once, especially when they are consumed along with other FODMAP foods.

~ ~ ~

A FODMAP elimination diet must be administered by a dietitian with experience in this type of diet approach. The first step is to eliminate all foods that contain FODMAPs for a trial period of around one to two weeks. If FODMAP carbs are indeed causing your symptoms, you will find relief in just a few days. FODMAP carbs are slowly and individually added back to your diet, one at a time, to find out which ones are causing problems and which ones are well-tolerated. The goal is to eliminate only the types of FODMAP carbs that cause symptoms so that you can follow a liberal and varied diet. Even if a FODMAP is found to cause problems, many people can still tolerate it in smaller doses. The FODMAP diet approach can be complicated, but if you are willing to try it, it can be quite useful in keeping your symptoms under control. To find more information on FODMAPs, visit: *http://blog.katescarlata.com/fodmaps-basics/fodmaps-checklist/*.

chapter 3

your five-step nutrition and lifestyle solution

How you treat your body nutritionally and physically can have a massive impact on your gut health. Diets low in fiber and high in sugars and refined grains, excessive alcohol intake, antibiotics, acid-blocking medications, chronic stress, excess body weight, and a sedentary lifestyle are just some of the factors that can impact our gut flora in a negative way. Good digestive health is an essential key to better overall health. By initiating the following steps, not only will you begin to heal and protect your gut, but you will also impact your health in so many other positive ways. The best part is that all five of these steps are fairly simple to implement into your everyday life, and can provide you with the power to take control of your lifestyle and your health.

Step 1: Commit to Cleaner Eating

Many Americans deal with digestive issues such as IBS, acid reflux, ulcers, and so on, and this has much to do with the foods we eat on a regular basis. As Americans we tend to fill up on processed foods rather than enjoying foods in their natural state. "Cleaner" eating basically involves reducing the amount of processed foods you eat and eating more whole foods in the form of fruits, vegetables, nuts, seeds, and whole grains. This isn't a diet, but a lifestyle choice that can make a difference to your gut and your overall health, not to mention your weight! To be successful at modifying your diet for the long haul, make changes one at a time instead of trying to go full steam ahead and changing everything at once. Start with adding a few servings of fruit each day, then add vegetables. Swap out your daily soft drink(s) for water, and instead of chips, snack on fruit or nuts. It won't take long before your cravings for sugar, fat, and processed foods subside, and reaching for healthier alternatives becomes a habit. The easiest way to think about eating more cleanly is really about choosing healthier foods in general. Cleaner eating may take a little more planning ahead, preparation, and time, but the outcome will be more than worth the investment.

Your Nutrition Solution Tidbit: Cleaner eating is not about following a specific diet; rather, it's about cleaning up your current diet. Use the tips provided and make an effort to eat cleaner, fresher foods that will ultimately effect a positive change to your overall health *and* your gut.

Here are a few tips to help you commit to cleaner eating.

- **Eat five to six times per day.** Eat three moderate meals and two to three small snacks each day, every two to three hours. Include lean protein, fresh fruit and/or vegetables, and a complex carbohydrate, especially whole grains, with each meal. This helps to keep your body fueled and burning calories efficiently all day long. It also gives you more opportunities to include the foods you need daily, especially fruits and vegetables.

- **Include fruits and vegetables at each meal and in most snacks.** Whether fresh or frozen, fruits and vegetables are chock full of all of the essential nutrients we need for good health and an even healthier gut. Eat a variety of produce; if you only have a few types that you eat, it's time to broaden your horizons! Make it a goal to incorporate at least one new fruit or vegetable into your meals every few weeks. Be sure to cook your produce with no added fats and sauces, and don't overcook them. Overcooking vegetables can destroy nutrients and break down that much-needed fiber. Try lightly steaming them or roasting them under the broiler for a few minutes with just a touch of olive oil.

- **Opt for water.** Water is essential for the proper functioning of the body and can help with digestion, metabolism, energy levels, lubricating sore joints, appetite control, and so much more. Avoid beverages such as soft drinks that are high in calories and sugar and lacking nutrients. When choosing juice, look for "100% juice" on the label to be sure there are no added sugars. Keep in mind when you're eating healthier and adding high-fiber foods, you'll need to increase your water intake, too.

- **Get label savvy.** "Clean" foods should contain the least amount of ingredients. Any food product with a long list of ingredients—five or more, especially ones you have never heard of—are probably not "clean" or wholesome.

- **Reduce processed and refined grains and sugar.** These are found in foods such as white bread, pasta, sugary cereal, baked goods, and so on. The closer foods are to their natural state, the less processed they are and, therefore, the more nutrient dense and healthier they are.

- **Know thine enemies.** Avoid foods high in saturated and trans fat, fried foods, and anything high in refined sugar. Both saturated and trans fat have adverse effects on our health, especially heart health. Saturated fats are found primarily in animal-based foods such as meat, the skin on poultry, butter, and high-fat products. Many baked goods and fried foods contain large amounts of saturated fat, as well. Trans fat is created when a liquid vegetable oil is made more solid by the addition of hydrogen through a process called *hydrogenation*. Foods highest in trans fats include fried foods, commercially baked goods, certain margarines, fast food such as French fries, and some processed snack foods such as crackers and chips.

- **Consume healthier fats more often.** Include essential fatty acids, especially omega-3 fatty acids, daily in the form of fatty fish, especially salmon, herring, tuna, mackerel, and sardines. Omega-3 fatty acids can also be found in a variety of plant foods such as walnuts, soybeans, chia seeds, flaxseeds, pumpkin seeds, olive oil, and numerous nut oils (in the form of ALA, or alpha linolenic acid). These healthy fats have numerous health benefits.

- **Choose the right meat.** Opt for meat that is grass fed and/or locally sourced, which will usually be free of hormones, antibiotics, and additives. Make meat a side dish rather than the focal point of your meal, and choose lean chicken, turkey, pork, or heart-healthy fish over red meat more often. When choosing red meat, stick with leaner cuts.

- **Go organic or locally grown.** Choose organic produce and other organic foods as often as possible. If budget restraints don't allow this, make meat, eggs, dairy, and the "dirty dozen" your priority.

Your Nutrition Solution Tidbit: The Environmental Working Group has put together a list of 12 fruits and vegetables (called the "dirty dozen") that are the most contaminated with the highest pesticide residue. If you are not up for buying everything organic, they sugest at least buying the following in organic form:

- Peaches
- Apples
- Sweet bell peppers
- Celery
- Nectarines
- Strawberries
- Cherries
- Pears
- Grapes (imported)
- Spinach
- Potatoes
- Lettuce

The following 12 fruits and vegetables are the least contaminated:

- Onions
- Avocados
- Sweet corn (frozen)
- Pineapples

- Mangos
- Asparagus
- Sweet peas (frozen)
- Kiwi fruit
- Bananas
- Cabbage
- Broccoli
- Papaya

For more information, check out *www.ewg.org*.

- **Slow down and enjoy.** Don't rush through your meals. Slow down and savor the taste of whole foods, and chew your foods well for better digestion.
- **Take it to go.** Pack a lunch bag or small cooler for work lunches, outings, school, and so on, so that you are always prepared and have whole, healthy foods on hand when you are out and about.
- **Get the family involved.** Don't just do it for your gut: make it a family affair! Improve the quality of your family's life and health along with your own by committing to cleaner eating.

Your Nutrition Solution Tidbit: ChooseMyPlate.gov and the Dietary Guidelines for Americans are issued and updated jointly by the Department of Agriculture (USDA) and the Department of Health and Human Services

(HHS) every five years. Both guidelines work hand-in-hand to provide the most current, scientifically based advice for all Americans two years old and older. They are available for all Americans so that we can educate ourselves as to what good nutrition is and how we can make healthier choices. The newest set of Dietary Guidelines for Americans focus on three major goals that, taken together, emphasize a total lifestyle approach:

1. Balancing calories with physical activity to manage weight.

2. Consume more healthy foods such as fruits, vegetables, whole grains, fat-free and low-fat dairy products, and seafood.

3. Consume fewer foods with sodium (salt), saturated fat, trans fat, cholesterol, added sugar, and refined grains.

For more information, check out *www .choosemyplate.gov* and *www.cnpp.usda.gov/ DietaryGuidelines.*

Step 2: Boost Your Daily Fiber Intake

Commit to boosting your fiber intake with beans, nuts, seeds, whole grains, fruits, and vegetables, all of which will help to improve and maintain good digestive health. Consuming ample amounts of fiber daily has plenty of digestive benefits. It can help to ease and regulate bowel movements; relieve and prevent constipation and diarrhea; reduce your risk of diverticulitis, hemorrhoids, gallstones, and kidney stones; and possibly provide relief of symptoms caused by IBS. Many fiber-rich foods act as prebiotics and help feed the good bacteria and probiotics in your gut so that they can do their job more efficiently and protect your GI tract. Incorporating high-fiber foods into your daily diet has other health benefits, including lowering the risk for heart disease, stroke, and diabetes; helping prevent certain cancers, such as colon cancer; and aiding in weight loss and weight maintenance.

There is no doubt that Americans need to eat more fiber daily, both for better overall health and a healthier gut. According to the National Academy of Sciences Institute of Medicine, the daily adequate intake (AI) for women is as follows:

- 50 years and younger: 25 grams
- 51 years and older: 21 grams

The daily adequate intake (AI) for men is a bit higher:

- 50 years and younger: 38 grams
- 51 years and older: 30 grams.

The key to reaping all the benefits of fiber is to maintain a good combination of both the soluble and insoluble kind.

Your Nutrition Solution Tidbit: When you increase your daily fiber intake, do so slowly and gradually. Drink plenty of water, too. Don't try to fit all of your fiber needs for the day into one meal. Instead, spread it out throughout the day and eat fiber-rich foods at every meal and snack. These tips will help prevent digestive discomfort as your body adjusts to this dietary change.

Here are some tips to help you boost your daily fiber intake:

- Start each day with a dose of fiber. Look for whole-grain cereals and whole-grain breads. You can add an additional 6 grams of fiber or more to your daily diet simply by switching your breakfast cereal.

- Add fruit to your breakfast meal. All fruit is a great source of fiber but in varying amounts.

- Keep plenty of fresh fruits and vegetables at your disposal. Wash and cut fruit and veggies and put them in air-tight containers in the refrigerator for quick and healthy snacks and for adding them to meals.

- Eat whole fruits and vegetables as opposed to drinking their juices. Whole fruits have much more fiber than their juice counterparts.

- Eat the skins of fruits and vegetables whenever possible, as that is where a lot of the fiber can be found, especially insoluble fiber. Examples include potatoes, apples, pears, and cucumbers. Note that some people with IBS and other digestive disorders may have a hard time digesting the skins. Eat them only if you can tolerate them, but if they cause discomfort, be sure to peel your fruits and vegetables.

Your Nutrition Solution Tidbit: According to the Dietary Guidelines for Americans you should be shooting for at least 2 1/2 cups of fruits and vegetables daily. Not only will they boost your fiber intake, but they will increase your intake of all types of vitamins, minerals, and other disease-fighting nutrients.

Add extra vegetables to dishes when cooking. Add them to soups, casseroles, stews, and stir-fries or mash them up and add them to thicken sauces or in mashed potatoes. Try using thinly sliced zucchini in place of lasagna noodles. Use your imagination and you will be shocked at how easy and tasty it can be to add more vegetables—and fiber—to your diet.

Snacks are a great place to add fiber to your day. In addition to fruits and vegetables as snack ideas, try dried fruits, whole-grain crackers, and nuts and seeds; or, whip up a smoothie that incorporates fresh fruits and/or vegetables.

Add ground flaxseed to yogurt, smoothies, oatmeal, applesauce, and breakfast cereals. Flax is a great source of fiber and also provides heart-healthy omega-3 fatty acids.

We all know what they say about beans, but did you know what a great source of fiber they are? Beans and peas are actually legumes, and include garbanzo beans (chickpeas), lima beans, pinto beans, cannellini beans, kidney beans, soybeans, great northern beans, black beans, fava beans, black-eyed peas, split peas, and lentils. The variety is endless. In addition to being rich in fiber they are also excellent sources of protein, iron, zinc, potassium, and folate. Legumes are incredibly versatile: You can add them to casseroles, stews, soups, salads, tacos—almost any of your favorite recipes.

> **Your Nutrition Solution Tidbit:** When you are looking to boost your fiber intake, food claims can make it a bit easier. Look for the following package claims when opting for higher fiber foods:
>
> **"Good source" of fiber** = the product contains 10 percent or more of your daily dose of fiber (about 2.5 grams per serving).
>
> **"Rich in," "high in," "excellent source of"** = the product contains 20 percent or more of your daily dose of fiber (about 5 grams per serving).

Fiber supplements

Hands down, the best way to get your daily intake of fiber is through foods that are naturally rich in fiber, as we've already discussed. However, if that proves difficult, taking a fiber supplement can help you to fill the gap and meet your daily requirement. The key is to get as much of your fiber through food as possible, and to use a supplement to do just that: *supplement* your fiber intake. Never let a fiber supplement take the place of whole foods, because these foods also contain loads of essential nutrients that you would otherwise be missing out on.

Fiber supplements come in a variety of forms, the most popular being chewable tablets or powders that you dissolve in water or add to foods. They are commonly made from "functional" fiber. (While dietary fiber comes from non-digestible carbs, and is intrinsic in plants, functional fiber comes from isolated or purified carbs.) Some of the best fiber supplements for gut health include:

- **Inulin and oligofructose (fructans)** are prebiotic ingredients that help encourage the growth of the beneficial bacteria in the gut, which helps to improve immunity and GI health.

- **Psyllium** is a type of soluble fiber that is effective in treating constipation and helping to relieve some symptoms of IBS.

- **Acacia fiber** is a type of soluble fiber that has been found to aid in the treatment of digestive disorders, especially IBS.

Fiber supplements can be a helpful addition to a healthy, fiber-rich diet; however it is possible to overdo a good thing. Taking excess fiber supplements can cause uncomfortable side effects such as diarrhea, gas, bloating, and abdominal discomfort. In addition, excess fiber can bind to iron, zinc, calcium, and magnesium, thus impeding their absorption in the body. To help ward off these unwanted side effects, don't take more fiber than you need, gradually increase the amount you take each day, drink plenty of liquids throughout the day, and spread the fiber throughout the day so you are not taking it all in one sitting. Fiber supplements can also interact with some medications such as antidepressants, cholesterol-lowering medications, and anticoagulant drugs, so check with your doctor before starting a fiber supplement regimen. Take your fiber supplement separately from medications, including over-the-counter vitamins and minerals, and take medications at least one hour before or two hours after the fiber supplement for optimal results.

Step 3: Limit Added Sugar

It is all too easy to overdo your sugar intake. According to a report from the 2005–2010 NHANES (National Health and Nutrition Examination Survey) database, Americans consume an average of about 20 teaspoons of sugar per day, with teens and men consuming the most. We are not talking about the natural sugar found in foods such as fruit and milk, but the added sugar that we really don't need. The majority of sugar found in the average American diet is added sugar. This sugar is added in processing, preparation, or at the table to sweeten and improve palatability. It is also added as a preservative and to provide texture, body, viscosity, and browning capacity to foods. Although the human body can't tell the difference between natural and added sugars, foods containing natural sugar usually contain the whole package of nutrients and other healthful components, such as fiber, that can slow down the absorption of sugar into the bloodstream. Most foods with added sugar often supply calories with little to no essential nutrients and no fiber.

Your Nutrition Solution Tidbit: If you are consuming a small amount of added sugar, such as choosing a flavored yogurt or adding a bit of sugar to a whole grain cereal, to improve the taste and acceptance of a healthier food, than that is an acceptable use of added sugars opposed to eating foods that are highly sweetened and contain absolutely no nutritional value.

What does sugar mean for the gut? Excess amounts of sugar encourage bad gut bacteria to reproduce, flourish, and overwhelm the GI tract, making less room for the "good" or "friendly" bacteria. We learned in Chapter 2 that added sugar most definitely does more harm than good for the digestive system, our weight, and our overall health. The American Heart Association recommends that Americans use no more than half of their daily discretionary calorie allowance for added sugars. For most women this would be no more than 100 calories per day, or about 6 teaspoons. For most men this would be no more than 150 calories per day, or about 9 teaspoons. Just to help put this in perspective, an average 12-ounce can of soda has around 8 to 10 teaspoons of sugar; and a breakfast cereal with 16 grams of sugar per serving contains about 4 teaspoons of sugar. One teaspoon of sugar is equal to about 4 grams of sugar.

Your Nutrition Solution Tidbit: *Discretionary calories* are basically calories that the body doesn't need to function. How many discretionary calories a person can eat without gaining weight depends on his or her physical activity and how many calories his or her body needs to meet daily nutritional requirements. Depending on the foods that you choose and how much physical activity you engage in daily, you may have more calories "left over" to spend on extras, including foods that contain added sugar. Although considered "extra," they should still be spent wisely. Other discretionary calories are often consumed in the form of fats, oils, and alcohol.

It isn't always easy to lower your intake of added sugar. The craving for sugar can be like an addiction for some people, and it takes time to change that sweet-tooth behavior. But the results will be positive ones, including everything from a healthier gut and weight loss to lowering your risk for heart disease. You don't need to completely eliminate all sugar from your diet, but you should keep it to a minimum. Here are a few tips to help you start to limit your sugar intake:

- When that sweet tooth hits, grab something with natural sugar and good nutritional value such as fruit, low-fat yogurt, or fat-free milk.

- When your craving for sweets takes over, try keeping yourself busy with something else such as taking a quick walk for a good 10 minutes. Many times cravings will disappear if you can distract yourself long enough.

- Be careful of foods that state they are "sugar-free" on the label. They may have low or no sugar, but the resulting "flavor gap" is often filled with fat. Read labels and watch your calorie intake.

- If you have a soft drink addiction, now is the time to change that. Soda is loaded with simple sugars and calories, and has absolutely no nutritional value. Try to slowly replace one can per week with water. Continue to slowly decrease the amount of soda you consume until you are either not drinking it anymore or drinking it only for special occasions.

- If you are a coffee or tea drinker, watch the amount of sugar you add to your cup. If you drink enough cups during the day, the sugar can add up quickly.

- Keep a pack of sugar-free gum on hand and enjoy a piece when you get the urge for something sweet.

- When you eat something sweet, watch your serving size and go ahead and enjoy it, but only on occasion.

- Choose your breakfast cereal carefully. You may think you are doing a good thing by choosing a whole-grain cereal, but don't forget to check the sugar content. A little bit to make it tastier is fine, but keep an eye on serving size. Skip the non-nutritious, sugary, and frosted cereals altogether.

- Most of all, be realistic. You can't stay away from your favorite sweets forever! But you can greatly reduce your intake of these added sugars and save these foods for an occasional treat instead of having them as a regular part of your daily diet.

Identifying added sugar

Identifying how much added sugar is in a food by using the food label can get tricky. When using the label to look for total number of grams of sugar per serving, you need to keep in mind that the sugar shown on the label represents both naturally occurring and added sugar. The only reliable way to identify added sugar in a product is to take a peek at the ingredient list. Ingredients are listed in descending order by weight. Look for sugar listed among the first few ingredients to determine if the product is high in added sugars. You won't always see the word "sugar" on the list, which makes it even harder to find it. Sugar can go by many different names, depending on its source and how it was made. Ingredients that end in "-ose" are the chemical names for the many types of sugar, including fructose, sucrose, maltose, glucose, lactose, and dextrose. Other common types of added sugar include cane sugar/juice/syrup, corn sweetener, honey, malt syrup, molasses, syrup, high-fructose corn syrup, powdered sugar, raw sugar, beet sugar, invert sugar, and brown sugar.

Your Nutrition Solution Tidbit: Fruit juices seem like they should be healthy beverages, but beware: many can be quite high in added sugar. The percent of actual juice that is in a beverage can be found on the package's label. Unless a package states "100% juice," it is not 100-percent juice. That means the product is a sweetened juice product with minimal juice content and added sugars. Avoid beverages that are labeled as "drinks" or "from concentrate," as they usually contain little to no juice and are loaded with sugar.

Step 4: Opt for Whole Grains

When whole grains are refined, essential vitamins, minerals, and dietary fiber are removed in the process. Many times these processed or refined grains are enriched with iron, thiamin, riboflavin, niacin, and folic acid before they are used as ingredients in foods. This enrichment process only returns some of the nutrients that were removed during refining. When consumed in excess, especially when they take the place of whole grains, processed grains commonly provide excess calories as well as added sugar and unhealthy added fat. With the lack of fiber, the health of our gut suffers. Fiber is what helps sweep the gut clean and supports the vitally important elimination and detoxification processes. In addition, refined grains release sugar rapidly, which is also tough on the gut and digestion.

Your Nutrition Solution Tidbit: According to the Dietary Guidelines for Americans, on average, Americans consume a little more than 6 ounces of refined grains per day. For a 2,000 calorie diet, the recommended amount of refined grains is no more than 3 ounces per day.

Swap whole grains for refined grains

Refined grains can be found in a lot of the foods Americans typically eat, including white bread, tortillas, bagels, pizza, white rice, pasta, cookies, cakes, donuts, and other desserts, just to name a few. Swapping these foods for whole grains is a small change that can make a big difference, both in keeping your gut healthy and managing and treating your symptoms of GI disorders. Upping your whole-grain intake as well as decreasing your refined grain intake are both part of the U.S. Dietary Guidelines for Americans. The current Dietary Guidelines for Americans recommends that adults eat at least half of their grains as whole grains. That adds up to at least three to five servings of whole grains daily.

Examples of one serving of whole grains:

- 1 slice whole-wheat bread
- 1 cup ready-to-eat whole-grain cereal
- 1/2 cup oatmeal
- 1/2 cup brown or wild rice
- 1/2 whole-grain English muffin
- 3 cups plain popcorn
- 1/2 cup whole-grain pasta

Whole grains include wheat, rye, spelt, rice, corn, and oats, and are found in foods such as oatmeal, brown rice, wild rice, popcorn, whole-wheat flour, bran, whole-grain couscous, whole-grain cereals and breads, and whole-grain pasta. Here are a few more varieties of whole grains that you may not even know about:

- **Amaranth** has one of the highest levels of complete (high quality) protein of all the grains. It is gluten-free and popular in cereals, breads, muffins, crackers, and pancakes.

- **Barley** has a tough hull or outer coating, which makes it difficult to remove without losing some of the bran, which is an important part of a whole grain. Hulled barley retains more of the whole-grain nutrients but takes a long time to cook. Hull-less brands of barley are becoming more widely available. Lightly pearled barley is not a true whole grain, because small amounts of the bran are missing, but it is still high in fiber and healthier than a refined grain. When buying barley, look for whole barley, hulled barley, or hull-less barley to ensure it is a whole grain. Barley is often used in soups, as a side dish, or made into porridge. This grain is also extremely effective in lowering cholesterol.

- **Buckwheat** is not truly a grain, and is not even a wheat, as it technically comes from the family of the rhubarb. However, due to its nutritional content, nutty flavor, and appearance, it has been adopted into the grain family. Buckwheat is used in pancake mixes, soba noodles, crepes, and kasha. It is the only grain known to include a high level of a powerful antioxidant known as *rutin*, which has been shown to improve circulation and prevent LDL (the "bad" cholesterol) from obstructing blood vessels.

- **Bulgur** is often made from durum wheat although bulgur can be made from just about any type of wheat. Bulgur comes dried so needs to be cooked before eating but it only takes about 10 minutes. This whole grain has a mild flavor and is often used as a side dish, pilaf, in salads, or in a popular dish known as tabbouleh. Bulgur is extremely high in fiber, in fact it has more than other whole grains including quinoa, oats, millet, buckwheat, and corn.

- **Millet** is versatile grain that can be used in everything from flatbreads to porridges as well as side dishes and desserts. Millet can be used in its whole form or ground into flour. This whole grain is gluten-free, easy to prepare, and has a delicate flavor. Millet is naturally high in protein content as well as antioxidants and can be very helpful in controlling blood sugar and blood cholesterol levels.

- **Quinoa** (pronounced "keen-wah") makes an easy, tasty, and healthy side dish. It cooks quickly and can also be used in soups, salads, and baked goods. Always be sure to rinse your quinoa before cooking. This grain is an excellent source of high-quality, complete protein as well as fiber.

- **Teff** is a type of millet that has a very small grain. It has a sweet flavor that is versatile for cooking, often used as porridge or added to baked goods. Teff has twice as much iron as most other grains and three times the calcium.

*To learn more about whole grains and try new recipes, visit: http://wholegrainscouncil.org.

Here are some easy tips for switching to whole grains:

- Try rolled oats, steel-cut oats, barley, buckwheat, or other whole grains as a hot breakfast cereal in place of refined white toast or a sugary cereal.

- Substitute half of the refined flour for whole-wheat flour in your baked goods. You can even try adding up to 20 percent of another whole-grain flour such as sorghum. You can try whole grain flour as a thickener when a recipes calls for it.

- Step up your breakfast foods by making pancakes or muffins using a combination of whole-grain flours instead of all refined white flour.

- Choose whole-grain bread, buns, rolls, pitas, English muffins, and bagels in place of those made with refined white flour.

- Try brown rice, wild rice, whole-grain couscous, barley, or bulgur in place of white rice as a side dish or in recipes.

- Choose whole-grain pasta or one that is a blend of whole and refined grains, instead of refined white pasta, with your favorite sauces or in casseroles, soups, and cold salads.

- Add cooked bulgur, brown or wild rice, whole-grain couscous, or barley to your favorite canned or homemade soup for an instant serving or more of whole grains.

- Jazz up your holiday bread stuffing with cooked bulgur, wild rice, or barley.

- Add three-quarters of a cup of uncooked oats to each pound of ground turkey or chicken breast to make meatballs, stuffed peppers, burgers, or meatloaf. This adds flavor and makes a great meat extender.

- Stir a handful of rolled oats into your favorite low-fat yogurt.

- Use oat bran to coat fish or chicken in place of refined bread crumbs.

- Look for snack foods, such as chips, that are made with whole grains.

How to find whole grains

You want to switch to eating more whole grains and weeding out the refined grains, but how do you know what foods are and are not made with whole grains? The whole grain stamp from the Whole Grains Council makes it easier than you think. There actually two different stamps that you will see on packaged foods:

The 100% stamp means that all of the grains in the product are whole grains and that there is a minimum of 16 grams (a full serving) of whole grains per labeled serving.

The basic stamp means that the product contains at least 8 grams (a half serving) of whole grains per labeled serving, but that the product may also contain some refined grains. Even if a product contains larger amounts of whole grains, it will use the basic stamp if it contains any refined grains at all.

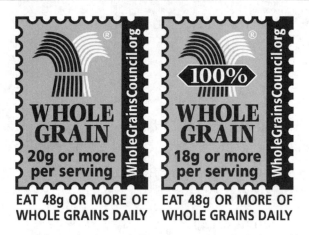

Because the whole grain stamp is not yet on all packaged foods, you still need to be aware of what to look for on labels. If there is no stamp, you can look for wording on the label that might state something like "100% whole wheat," which is a statement you can trust. But if you see something like "whole grain" without a little more explanation, this can mean that the food only contains a small amount of whole grains, so you might need to investigate a bit further. Check the ingredient list. If the first ingredient listed contains the word "whole"— such as "whole-wheat flour"—then it's likely that the food is made primarily with whole grains. If two flours are listed and only the second one states "whole," the product could contain anywhere from 1 to 49 percent whole grains.

The following words on a label mean that you are getting a whole grain:

- "Whole grain," "whole wheat," "whole [other grain]"

- "Stoneground whole [grain]"
- "Brown rice"
- "Wheatberries"
- "Oats," "oatmeal"

The following words on a label mean that the food is most likely missing some part of the whole grain:

- "Wheat" or "wheat flour"
- "Semolina"
- "Durum wheat"
- "Organic flour"
- "Stoneground"
- "Multigrain"

The following words on a label mean that the food is definitely *not* a whole grain:

- "Enriched flour"
- "Degerminated corn meal"
- "Bran"
- "Wheat germ"

The key is to find ways to fit whole grains into your diet anywhere you can. Remember that a little bit can go a long way but shoot for as many as you can. Always check food labels and ingredient lists to ensure you are actually buying a whole grain product. Continue to gather information about whole grains and the vast variety that is out there to try.

Step 5: Reach and Maintain a Healthy Weight

In addition to all of the general health risks that obesity sets you up for, such as heart disease, diabetes, and hypertension, obesity is associated with a number of health issues that affect your digestive system. GI diseases are two to three times more likely in those who are obese than those who are at a healthy weight. Being overweight or obese puts you at a higher risk for acid reflux, Barrett's esophagus, cancer of the esophagus, precancerous and cancerous polyps in the colon, gallstones, acute pancreatitis, cancer of the gallbladder and pancreas, and various liver diseases. When high levels of body fat are combined with physical inactivity, poor nutrition, and advanced age, the risk of gut disorders is increased even further. The good news is that making lifestyle changes, including weight loss, can help to reverse this. Losing just 10 percent of your current body weight can begin to reduce your risk for many health conditions, including GI conditions. If you are already at a healthy weight, the goal is to maintain that weight. If you are overweight or obese, the goal is to slowly and steadily lose weight in a healthy manner (no more than one or two pounds per week), until you reach a healthy weight. Always check with your doctor first to discuss the weight-loss strategy that is best for you and to be thoroughly checked out before starting any type of weight loss plan.

Your Nutrition Solution Tidbit: Several studies show the flip side of the weight coin. The overgrowth and imbalance of "unfriendly" bacteria in the gut may create leptin-resistant (leptin is an appetite hormone) and insulin-resistant obesity. (Source: Richards, Byron J. "How Imbalanced Digestive Bacteria Cause Obesity and Heart Disease." *Wellness Resources*, published May 20, 2013. Webpage accessed January 21, 2015.) This is yet another very good reason to ensure you have a healthy gut and healthy gut flora.

Determine your healthy weight

Let's say you have determined that you need to lose weight. The question is, how much? How can you find out what your healthy weight should be? The body mass index (BMI) is one way to determine whether your extra pounds translate into greater health risks, including the risk for gut disorders. BMI is the measurement of your weight relative to your height and can determine whether you are at a healthy weight or if your weight is possibly contributing to poor health and an unhealthy gut. Keep in mind that BMI is not a measurement of body fat; therefore it can sometimes misclassify people. For example, people with a lot of muscle mass may have a BMI that registers as too high, because BMI doesn't take into consideration that most of their body weight is coming from muscle, not fat. It can do the opposite for elderly people and underestimate BMI, not taking into account the muscle mass they have lost through the years. However, for the majority of us, BMI is a good general indicator of what our healthy weight range should be and whether we are putting ourselves at risk for health issues related to our weight.

You can crunch the numbers yourself by using this formula:

Weight in pounds ÷ [height in inches] squared x 703

You can also find calculators online such as this one: *www.choosemyplate.gov/supertracker-tools/resources/bmi-calculator.html.* Or, you can use the chart* below to easily find your BMI:

BMI	19	20	21	22	23	24	25	26	27	28	29	30	31	32	33	34	35
Height								Weight in Pounds									
4'10"	91	96	100	105	110	115	119	124	129	134	138	143	148	153	158	162	167
4'11"	94	99	104	109	114	119	124	128	133	138	143	148	153	158	163	168	173
5'	97	102	107	112	118	123	128	133	138	143	148	153	158	163	168	174	179
5'1"	100	106	111	116	122	127	132	137	143	148	153	158	164	169	174	180	185
5'2"	104	109	115	120	126	131	136	142	147	153	158	164	169	175	180	186	191
5'3"	107	113	118	124	130	135	141	146	152	158	163	169	175	180	186	191	197
5'4"	110	116	122	128	134	140	145	151	157	163	169	174	180	186	192	197	204
5'5"	114	120	126	132	138	144	150	156	162	168	174	180	186	192	198	204	210
5'6"	118	124	130	136	142	148	155	161	167	173	179	186	192	198	204	210	216
5'7"	121	127	134	140	146	153	159	166	172	178	185	191	198	204	211	217	223
5'8"	125	131	138	144	151	158	164	171	177	184	190	197	203	210	216	223	230
5'9"	128	135	142	149	155	162	169	176	182	189	196	203	209	216	223	230	236
5'10"	132	139	146	153	160	167	174	181	188	195	202	209	216	222	229	236	243
5'11"	136	143	150	157	165	172	179	186	193	200	208	215	222	229	236	243	250
6'	140	147	154	162	169	177	184	191	199	206	213	221	228	235	242	250	258
6'1"	144	151	159	166	174	182	189	197	204	212	219	227	235	242	250	257	265
6'2"	148	155	163	171	179	186	194	202	210	218	225	233	241	249	256	264	272
6'3"	152	160	168	176	184	192	200	208	216	224	232	240	248	256	264	272	279
6'4"	156	164	172	180	189	197	205	213	221	230	238	246	254	263	271	279	287
	Healthy Weight						Overweight					Obese					

*Source: Evidence Report of Clinical Guidelines on the Identification, Evaluation, and Treatment of Overweight and Obesity in Adults, 1998. NIH/National Heart, Lung, and Blood Institute (NHLBI). For additional heights and weights visit: www.nhlbi.nih.gov/guidelines/obesity/bmi_tbl.htm.

To use this BMI chart, locate your height in the left-hand column and follow the row across that height to find your weight. Follow that column of the weight up to the top to locate your BMI. Now that you know your BMI, what exactly does it mean? Healthy weight is a range and not one single weight. The following will show you what range you fall into and what your BMI means for you:

BMI	Weight
Below 18.5	Underweight
18.5 to 24.9	Healthy Weight
25.0 to 29.9	Overweight
Over 30.0	Obese

Take the weight off for good

We have learned that an unhealthy gut can lead to weight gain, and that excess weight can lead to an unhealthy gut. So, in addition to taking steps to increase your gut health, you should also be taking steps to reach a healthy weight. If you have a long way to go before you get to your healthy weight range, take heart knowing that even a little bit of effort can go a long way. If you are on the overweight side of the coin, losing just five to 10 percent of your current weight can sometimes be just the ticket to begin improving any weight-related conditions and your overall health. But don't stop there! Reaching your healthy weight once and for all will not only help to get your health under control, but it will most likely end up helping you in ways you never imagined.

Resist the urge to sign up for fad diets or any type of diet that promises quick and easy weight loss. These types of diets usually involve extreme deprivation, which can easily deplete your body's stores of essential nutrients. Not to mention that losing weight too quickly is usually the weight loss that never sticks. Steer clear of liquid diets, diet pills, or diet supplements that promise that tempting quick fix. Slow and steady wins the race to long lasting weight loss, a healthier gut, and better overall health. Losing one to two pounds per week is a safe and effective goal. The ultimate goal should to lose the weight and keep it off for good.

In order to begin losing weight, it doesn't take as much change as you might think. You can do it safely by subtracting as little as 250 to 500 calories per day. That can be as simple as eliminating a regular can of soda and that mid-day candy bar; we know that neither does your gut any good anyhow! There is no need to drastically change your entire diet all at once; instead make changes and cut back slowly. Making healthier choices by eliminating unhealthy foods and replacing them with healthier foods, such as the ones we've already talked about (whole grains, fruits, vegetables, nuts, seeds, lean meats, fish, and fat-free dairy products), will usually cut calorie intake automatically. As you lose weight and your body becomes accustomed to this new calorie level—which you might notice by experiencing a weight plateau—it may be time to make a few more changes and cut back a bit more. For permanent weight loss, you'll want to lose weight slowly, steadily, and in a healthy manner. It doesn't take a whole lot to begin reversing the process and getting yourself on track.

> **Your Nutrition Solution Tidbit:** About 3,500 calories add up to one pound. Therefore to lose one pound per week you need to split up a deficit of 3,500 calories over a week's time. Depending on your activity level and metabolism, deducting 500 calories per day should result in a weight loss of one pound per week.

The key is to worry less about every little calorie and concentrate more on eating nutrient- and fiber-rich foods that make each calorie count while still keeping an eye on your portion sizes. This will keep control of your calorie intake and ensure that even though you are trying to lose weight, you will still be getting all of the essential nutrients your body needs for good health. It's time to change bad habits into good ones and that goes for eating as well as exercise. Here are just a few strategies that may help you begin losing weight in a way that is healthy and optimizes your gut health:

- Your first order of business should be to consider your reasons for wanting to lose weight. Because you're already reading this book, it's a good bet that preventing and/or reducing symptoms of gut-related issues without the need for numerous and long-term medications will be somewhere on that list. Knowing exactly what will motivate you and keep you committed to your goals is what will ultimately make you successful in your endeavor! To stay committed, write down your goals and look at them whenever you need motivation.

- Set both short-term and long-term goals. Short-term goals are essential to keep you going on the journey to reach your long-term goal of a healthy weight. Your goals need to be realistic, specific, and measurable. Write them down, along with your motivations, so you always know what you are working toward. Don't expect to change *all* of your bad habits, or the habits that have caused that extra weight gain, all at one time. Work on changing habits a few at a time. Once you have mastered one goal, move on to the next.

- Keep a daily food diary that includes what you eat, when you eat, and how much you eat. Write it all down or find a free online food diary such as the Food Tracker on ChooseMyPlate.gov or a good app on your phone. Review your food diary frequently so that you can pinpoint and work on problem areas. Keeping a food diary will help to keep you compliant and on track and may also point out trigger foods for digestive issues.

- Be aware of everything you eat and drink. Make yourself accountable for what you eat and the way you live your life. Concentrate on eating for true hunger and for properly fueling your body, and not because you are emotional, stressed, or bored.

- Do not skip meals. This includes breakfast! Skipping a meal will not save calories and will only lead to eating more then you should at the next meal and/or cause uncontrolled snacking, usually on unhealthy foods. Eating a well-balanced healthy breakfast is associated with better weight loss and control throughout the rest of the day.

- Stick to a well-balanced and healthy eating routine. Healthier choices usually mean fewer calories, less fat, less sodium, and more nutritional value.

- Cut out your junk foods such as candy, cookies, cake, pies, other sweets, soft drinks, fast foods, and chips. Occasionally is okay, but indulging more often causes weight gain and can wreak havoc on gut health.

- Plan your healthy meals and snacks ahead of time so that you are always prepared.

- Include plenty of fiber in your diet daily. You already know that a diet rich in fiber can help decrease the risk of gut issues in addition to being very helpful with weight loss. High-fiber meals and snacks help fill you up and keep you feeling fuller longer. Check back to page 86 in this chapter for tips on how to incorporate more fiber in your diet.

- Keep your portions moderate and don't eat past the point of fullness. Eat until you are comfortable, not stuffed.

- Avoid eating in front of the television or while doing other activities that keep you from paying attention to how much you are eating.

- Eat more slowly. Chewing your food more thoroughly will help slow you down and is important for better digestion and gut health. It takes a good 20 minutes for your brain to get the message that you are full. Eating too quickly leads to overeating, excess weight, and digestive issues.

- Use a smaller plate to keep your portions and calories under control and make you feel that you are getting a full plate of food. Just don't go back for seconds!

- Plan and prepare meals at home to keep from eating out too often. Restaurant meals tend to be higher in calories, fat, and sodium, and it can be tempting to make the wrong choices when eating out. Don't completely deprive yourself of the treat of eating out, but make it an occasional venture instead of a regular habit, and make better choices when you do eat out.

- Learn how to read and use the nutrition facts panel on food labels to your advantage. The panel will help you choose foods that best fit into your goals. It will also help you assess portion sizes and calorie intake. We will discuss food labels in greater depth in Chapter 5.

- Check out the USDA's ChooseMyPlate.gov site to explore all of the information and hands-on tools that can help you lose weight sensibly and learn what good nutrition really means.

- Stay active. Incorporate physical activity most days of the week. Overweight and obesity are direct results of an imbalance between the calories you take in and the calories you burn. It is just that simple. The more active you are, the more calories you will burn.

- Drink plenty of water throughout the day, every day. Staying well-hydrated is essential to proper digestion and aids in fat burning.

If you need more personal guidance, and many people do, turn to a registered dietitian nutritionist (RDN) who can educate, guide, motivate, and keep you on track to future success. Check out *www.eatright.org* to find a dietitian in your area.

~ ~ ~

These simple tips and changes can help you improve your health, lose weight, and reduce gut symptoms. It is all about making permanent lifestyle changes. Once you begin to lose weight and feel better you will be motivated to push ahead and finish your journey.

Other Gut-Favorable Lifestyle Changes

Get your body moving

Getting your body moving every day can significantly aid in digestion and gut health. Being physically active on a regular basis may encourage the beneficial gut bacteria to thrive, whereas being physically inactive does the opposite. Exercise can boost the immune system, lower inflammation, balance hormones, aid in weight loss, increase heart health, better control blood sugar, improve sleep patterns, lower stress, and increase the motility of the bowels.

Exercise is more than cardiovascular fitness, and it certainly doesn't have to mean long hours at the gym. Exercise can be anything that helps to get your body moving. The goal is to get active and stay active on a regular basis with a solid exercise plan that fits you and your lifestyle. Exercise is one lifestyle change that has a direct correlation with better health in all studies. The key is to start moving and stay moving!

Your Nutrition Solution Tidbit: According to the Dietary Guidelines for Americans, adults aged 18 to 64 years should engage in at least two hours and 30 minutes (or 150 minutes) of aerobic activity at a moderate level each week; or one hour and 15 minutes (or 75 minutes) of aerobic physical activity at a vigorous level each week. Being active five or more hours weekly can provide even greater health benefits. Spreading your exercise over at least three days is suggested, and each activity should be done for at least 10 minutes at a time. Adults should also engage in resistance/strength training activities such as push-ups, sit-up and/ or lifting weights, at least 2 days per week.

With all of the benefits right there in front of you, it is pretty hard to say no to exercise. For some of us, though, it still takes a bit of motivation to get started and, especially, to stick with it. Here are a few tips to help you do just that:

- Don't go all out, right out of the gate; this can set you up for failure. Instead, start by setting one small, specific, and attainable goal; once you reach that goal, set a new one.

- Keep yourself motivated by the way you feel. Losing weight and simply feeling better physically can sometimes be all the motivation you need. Take note of weight loss and other positives such as feeling better both mentally and physically, feeling less fatigued, experiencing fewer GI symptoms, less pain in joint areas, and sleeping better through the night.

- Do activities you enjoy. Exercise doesn't necessarily mean hours at the gym (although some people love that!). It simply means getting your body moving at a good pace on a regular basis. Try swimming, dancing, tennis, walking, jogging, running, skiing, yoga, spinning, biking, hiking, horseback riding— whatever you enjoy!

- Schedule your daily exercise on your weekly calendar, just as you do for all your other weekly activities.

- Use visual cues as reminders and motivators. Stick a note on the refrigerator or your computer; put your workout shoes by the door that you always use.

- Get a workout buddy and do it together. Being accountable to another person is a huge motivator.

- Before you start exercising, whether you have never exercised before or are an avid exerciser, it is always smart to speak with your doctor about what is safe for you and your individual situation. It is important to have a few guidelines and warnings under your belt before you do get started.

- Aim for 30 minutes of moderate-to-vigorous intensity aerobic activity, at least five days per week, for a total of 150 minutes per week.

- Aim for strength training at least two times per week in addition to your aerobic exercise.

- If you have never exercised before, start slowly and work your way up. Start with five to 10 minutes a day and work up from there. Always begin by warming up, too. Your fitness will improve over time, and you will be able to do more for a longer period before you know it.

- For consistency, spread your physical activity out during the week so that you are able to exercise most days. Try to not go more than two days in a row without exercising.

- If you can't find the time for a block of 30 minutes, split it up into three 10-minute increments throughout your day.

- Eat a light snack about 30 minutes before you exercise. Something small with at least 30 grams of carbs and some protein will suffice. Try half a whole-grain bagel with peanut butter, or a banana and a handful of nuts. This will help fuel your workout.

- Drink plenty of water before, during, and after exercise.

- No matter what kind of activity you choose, always warm up for at least five minutes before starting your exercise and cool down for five minutes afterward. The best type of exercise program combines both aerobic and strength training.

Here are some other ideas to help you keep yourself moving all day long, even when you're not at the gym:

- Take the stairs instead of the elevator.

- Park at the far end of the parking lot for a longer walk (but be safe).

- Forget the drive-thru at the bank or the pharmacy; park and walk in instead.

- If you have a sit-down job, get up every 30 minutes or so and move around.

- Play actively with your kids instead of watching them from the sidelines.

- Take the dog for regular walks.

- Wash the car yourself instead of taking it to the car wash.

- When you're on the phone, walk around the house instead of sitting on the couch.

- Mow the grass, rake the leaves, and work in the garden (if you're lucky enough to have one).

Manage your stress

Stress can be a major contributor to many health-related issues. In addition to the personal stress of everyday life, our body experiences the stressors that come along with inadequate sleep, food sensitivities, environmental toxins, poor diets, and poor (or complete lack of) exercise habits. Besides impacting our emotional status, stress can affect our physical health and can be a main factor in poor gut health and functioning as well as an increased risk for chronic diseases. Stress can affect every aspect of the digestive system, causing digestive issues and making existing issues worse. When the body experiences stress, digestion can literally shut down due to the central nervous system's response. This in turn shuts down blood flow, which affects the muscles in the digestive tract and decreases the fluids needed for digestion. Stress can cause inflammation of the GI tract and make you more susceptible to infection, as well. Stress can cause spasms in your esophagus, increase stomach acid, and cause indigestion and acid reflux. It can cause nausea, diarrhea, and constipation. Although stress will not actually *cause* serious GI issues such as celiac disease, IBS, or IBD, it can contribute to flare-ups of symptoms.

Although we can't control or get rid of all the stressors in our life, we can learn to control and manage our stress better. Being stressed out from time to time is normal, but dealing with chronic stress on a daily basis can really do some damage. If you feel chronic stress is an issue for you, it is time to begin taking steps to learn some coping strategies that will help to decrease your stress levels before it does more physical damage.

Here are a few tips to help you out:

- Start a regular exercise program. This is a great stress reliever and, as an added bonus, can help you shed pounds.

- Write down your feelings and thoughts in a journal. Sometimes getting thoughts down on paper can get them off of your mind and help you to relax.

- Take a look at your daily schedule and see how you can start to slow down a bit by letting people help you with daily tasks.

- Meditate daily in a quiet area. Focus on the present and on your breathing. It can be tough at first, but you will eventually learn to shut everything out during that time and deeply relax.

- Try a meditative or relaxing type of yoga. Taking a class can help.

- Try getting regular massages.

- Look into alternative therapies such as acupuncture or Reiki therapy.

- Take up a new hobby that can be relaxing such as gardening, reading, working with animals, or whatever says "relax" to you.

- If you are unable to de-stress, speak with your doctor about a possible referral to a counselor who can help you out on a one-on-one basis.

chapter 4

10 foods to avoid and 10 foods to include for a healthier gut

Food has a lot to do with our GI tract and the health of the gut. The body will digest just about anything we put in our mouth, but that doesn't mean the GI tract will react well to everything we eat, nor does it mean we can easily digest all foods. We already know that highly processed foods, foods high in sugar and fat as well as fried foods can all spell trouble for our gut. We also know that fiber-rich foods and foods high in prebiotics and probiotics can benefit our gut. There isn't just one diet or one food that is the cure-all for our gut and gut issues; the key is to eat foods that nourish healthy gut bacteria and avoid foods that sustain harmful gut bacteria or harm the good bacteria. We will discuss some of these foods to give you an idea of foods to include and foods to avoid.

10 Foods to Avoid

We have discussed many components of foods that are known to hamper digestive health, including sugar, refined grains, and unhealthy fats. Whether you are already having digestive issues or not, what to avoid is just as important as what to include. Avoiding gut-busting foods may save you some GI troubles both now and down the road. Keep in mind that for some people, depending on their current GI disorder and/or food sensitivities or intolerances, specific foods may need to be avoided that would not normally be considered common digestive culprits. It is essential to know which foods affect you and your health the most and to ensure you avoid those foods. The following are some foods, beverages, and ingredients that can generally wreak havoc on your gut and digestive process and ones you should avoid whether you already have known digestive issues or not.

1. White bread

White bread is made with refined, white flour. Refined grains and the foods made with them—white bread, English muffins, bagels, white rice, and white pasta—are broken down rapidly into sugar in the digestive system. Sugar is damaging to the gut as it tends to destroy the "good" bacteria. In addition white bread has almost no fiber, which can lead to constipation in people who don't consume enough fiber daily. Eating too much white bread can actually lead to obesity, which in turn can lead to an unhealthy gut. Your best bet is choosing whole-wheat or whole-grain breads to boost your gut health and your overall health.

2. High-fructose corn syrup

Although all sugars will spike blood sugar, high fructose corn syrup (HFCS) is one to watch out for because it is added to so many foods and has some very negative implications for our gut and overall health. HFCS is an added sugar; the fructose from this sweetener requires additional energy from the gut for it to be absorbed properly. This takes up a lot of energy, leaving less available to help maintain the integrity of the intestinal lining. The result is leakage of bad gut bacteria through the cells of the intestinal walls, and partially digested food particles and toxic by-products triggering an immune reaction and chronic inflammation. This can become the root cause of obesity, cancer, heart disease, dementia, diabetes, and more. HFCS has also been linked to the increase of insulin resistance and triglycerides. HFCS represents more than 40 percent of the caloric sweeteners that are added to foods and beverages, and is the only caloric sweetener added to soft drinks in the United States. There is no way of knowing how much HFCS is in a food or beverage, but you can read the ingredient list on the food label to give you a clue. If HFCS is one of the first ingredients listed, it is safe to assume that the product contains quite a bit. Your best option is to check labels and avoid foods and beverages that contain any amount of HFCS. Avoiding highly processed foods and sticking with fresh, whole foods will not only benefit your gut but will help you to avoid HFCS. Common foods that contain HFCS include regular soft drinks, syrups, breakfast cereals, fruit juices, popsicles, fruit-flavored yogurts, ketchup, BBQ sauce, canned and jarred pasta sauce, canned soup, and canned fruit (if in syrup), just to name a few.

3. Alcohol

Regular excessive intake of alcoholic beverages can have many negative health effects, including chronic acid reflux, liver damage, heart disease, insulin resistance, esophageal cancer, poor nutritional intake, and gastric ulcers from increased acid production. More immediate symptoms can include heartburn, diarrhea, headache, constipation, and vomiting. Prolonged and heavy use of alcohol can wreak havoc all over your body by increasing the production of cytokines and other pro-inflammatory markers. It can disturb the intestinal absorption of nutrients, including many vitamins as well as sodium, potassium, and water. Dehydration causes your body to work overtime to recover fluids and electrolytes from anywhere it can get them, including your GI tract. This can cause constipation along with a nasty headache the next day. Excessive alcohol intake can lead to bleeding and injury to the walls of the intestines and an overgrowth of "bad" bacteria. The damage done to the inside walls of the digestive tract allows bacterial toxins to enter the blood, increasing the liver's exposure to toxins and thus increasing the risk of liver disease. Because heavy drinkers usually have higher levels of the stress-response hormone cortisol in their body than non-drinkers, they are more susceptible to depression, other addictions, and frequent mood changes. Moderate consumption of alcoholic beverages—one drink per day for women and two drinks per day for men—*may* have a few health benefits. But if you feel you are drinking too much, too often, see your doctor to start discussing ways you can take back control of your life and your health.

> **Your Nutrition Solution Tidbit:** One drink is equal to one 12-ounce beer, one 8-ounce glass of malt liquor, one 5-ounce glass of wine, or 1.5 ounces of 80-proof distilled spirits or liquor.

4. Coffee

Coffee is very much a part of many people's everyday routine. However, that coffee contains oils, acids, and caffeine that can irritate the lining of your stomach and small intestine. Consuming coffee causes an overproduction of hydrochloric acid (HCL) in your stomach, which can cause irritation, especially in someone who already suffers from a GI disorder. Coffee can exacerbate acid reflux and heartburn. For those suffering from IBS, gastritis, Crohn's disease, colitis, or ulcers, coffee can be a potent irritant. The specific type of acid content in coffee can actually create perfect conditions for *H. pylori* to flourish, which can lead to ulcers. Switching to decaf won't help, because it isn't the caffeine but rather the acids and enzymes in the coffee beans that cause the issues. The acidity in coffee—regular and decaf—can prevent healing of a GI tract that is already damaged. These same substances can have a severe laxative effect in some people. Caffeine acts as a diuretic, which can lead to the loss of essential nutrients such as vitamins and minerals, and even dehydration. Coffee doesn't need to be completely off the table if you suffer from GI disorders (unless, of course, you have been told by your doctor not to drink it). However, it should be consumed in moderation. Opting for water is always the safer and healthier route.

5. Fast food

Fast food can be detrimental to anyone's diet, but when it comes to gut health, these foods are toxic. They can make the digestive system sluggish, causing constipation and aggravating other GI disorders; or, they can move too quickly through the GI system, causing diarrhea. Additionally, they can cause indigestion, heartburn, bloating, and a feeling of over-fullness. Not only do most fast food meals contain loads of calories, which can lead to weight gain, but they are also loaded with sodium, cholesterol, trans fat, saturated fat, and refined grains. As well, they lack the fiber and essential nutrients that are so important to good gut health and healthy gut flora. Unhealthy and dangerous trans fats have been connected to esophageal disease and should be extremely limited in any diet. The problem is that most of us are busy people, and eating on the run is a convenient option. If you find yourself in this situation, the key is to make healthier choices and to not let yourself be tempted by the foods you know you should not have. Stay away from "super-sizing," and take a look at nutritional information, which all fast food places now provide, before you order. Avoid foods that are high in calories, bad fats, refined grains, sodium, and sugar, and chose healthier options such as fresh salad, fruit, grilled chicken, and anything made with whole grains. If you know you are going to be out and about, carry food with you and/or choose a fast food establishment where you know you can get healthier options. Fast food on occasion is one thing, but making it a regular habit can definitely lead to a host of health issues, including an unhealthy gut.

6 Soft drinks

Soft drinks (also called "soda" or "pop," depending on where you live), whether diet or full of sugar, seem to be the drink of choice for many Americans these days. Soft drinks are what we dietitians call "empty calories," meaning, these beverages provide calories but have absolutely no nutritional value. In addition to the adverse health effects that drinking too many soft drinks can lead to, going overboard can also be an easy way to put on the pounds, which can lead to an unhealthy gut. These types of beverages contain many other substances, none of them beneficial to your health. Most contain phosphoric acid, which has been shown to deplete calcium stores from our bones, leading to osteoporosis, weakened bones, and decreased bone mass. The average 12-ounce can of cola contains a whopping 9 teaspoons of refined sugar in the form of high-fructose corn syrup, which depletes healthy gut flora and nourishes the "bad" bacteria. The carbonation in soft drinks may cause belching, gas, and indigestion. And let's not forget the caffeine, especially in colas and energy drinks, which can cause intestinal upset due to its laxative effect on the GI tract. Caffeine can trigger the release of gastric juices and cause food to be transferred into the small intestines before they are fully digested. It can also cause the lower esophageal sphincter muscle to relax, resulting in acid reflux and heartburn. If you think switching to "diet" soft drinks will help you out, think again: Your best bet is to either avoid soft drinks altogether or at the least drink them only on occasion. Stick with water, fat-free dairy, or soy/nut beverages, 100-percent juices, or unsweetened hot or iced tea.

7. Artificial sweeteners

Just because the sugar has been taken out doesn't mean it's a healthy beverage. Diet soft drinks are made with artificial sweeteners, or sugar substitutes, which for some people can cause digestive symptoms such as gas and bloating. Researchers from Duke University published a study in the *Journal of Toxicology and Environmental Health* that explained that a specific artificial sweetener called Splenda may significantly decrease the number of good bacteria in the gut. (Source: Abou-Donia, M.B., El-Masry, E.M., et al. "Splenda Alters Gut Microflora and Increases Intestinal P-glycoprotein and Cytochrome P-450 in Male Rats." *Journal of Toxicology and Environmental Health* 71.21 (2008): 1415–429. National Center for Biotechnology Information, U.S. National Library of Medicine/PubMed. gov. Webpage accessed February 4, 2015.) Another study published in 2014 by Dr. Eran Elinay of the Weizmann

Institute of Science's Department of Immunology found that gut bacteria reacted to artificial sweeteners and promoted glucose intolerance in some people. (Source: Elinav, Eran. "Gut Bacteria, Artificial Sweeteners, and Glucose Intolerance." American Committee for the Weizmann Institute of Science. N.p., 17 Sept. 2014. Webpage accessed February 1, 2015.) Because artificial sweeteners are so much sweeter than regular sugar, researchers have found that consuming too many can overstimulate the sugar receptors. This causes people to find less sweet foods, such as fruit, not as appealing. This then tends to cause avoidance of healthy, filling, and highly nutritious foods and instead choosing artificially flavored foods with less nutritional value. As of this writing, much-needed research continues on the consumption of artificial sweeteners. So stay tuned.

Your Nutrition Solution Tidbit: Sugar alcohol is another type of low-calorie sweetener. It's often added to sugar-free foods such as chocolates, confections, gum, and mints. Because it is not easily digested it can produce gas, bloating, cramping, and diarrhea in some people. The American Dietetic Association warns that more than 50 grams of sorbitol or 20 grams of mannitol per day can cause diarrhea. People with GI issues are most at risk for the side effects of sugar alcohol, so check out the nutrition information label on sugar-free foods to know how much of this sweetener you are consuming.

8. Red meat

Who doesn't love a juicy burger or sizzling steak? Unfortunately, a diet heavy in red meat has long been tied to the increased risk for *atherosclerosis*, or hardening of the arteries. A study at the Cleveland Clinic found that a diet that includes red meat and carnitine (a compound found in red meat) can shift the composition of bacteria in our gut toward those that are more prone to promoting heart disease. (Source: Koeth, Robert, A., Zeneng Wang, et al. "Intestinal Microbiota Metabolism of L-carnitine, a Nutrient in Red Meat, Promotes Atherosclerosis." Nature Medicine 19 (2013): 576–85. Published April 7, 2013. Webpage accessed January 30, 2015.) Eating a diet that includes a lot of red meat can also increase your risk for colon cancer, because red meat is high in saturated fat. The solution is to decrease your intake of red meat as much as possible. Stick with chicken, poultry, fish/seafood, and lean cuts of pork, and eat leaner cuts of red meat only on occasion. Try other sources of protein, too, including soy, legumes/beans, lentils, egg whites, and peanut butter. Nothing wrong with making that juicy burger out of ground turkey breast or even a Portobello mushroom, or substituting that sizzling steak with a chunk of marinated salmon on the grill. Your gut and your heart will thank you for it!

9. Frozen dinners

Yes, they are convenient. Some may even seem healthy, but think again. Frozen dinners do have a few benefits, as they provide instant portion control and make for a quick and easy meal. However, most dinners are low in whole grains and produce and high in sodium whether you choose the lower fat and healthier versions or not. If you take a good look at the majority of them, they are highly processed, with all types of ingredients you won't recognize. And as we know, highly processed foods are a breeding ground for bad bacteria to flourish. Many of them contain ingredients it is best to stay away from for a healthier gut including high fructose corn syrup, trans fat (partially hydrogenated oil), saturated fat, and the list goes on. In addition, the majority of these meals do not contain whole grains, and the vegetable portions are quite small to say the least. As always, your best choice is to eat meals made from whole, fresh foods. Taking the time to make meals ahead can make eating whole, fresh foods much more convenient. If you find yourself in a hurry and need something fast, a healthier version of a frozen meal can be much better than the wrong choice at a fast food restaurant. Choosing a frozen meal on occasion won't destroy your gut, but you still need to keep some important guidelines in mind when choosing them:

- Select meals that have 350 to 500 calories for the entire meal. Anything lower than that, and you really aren't getting enough food to provide any substantial amount of energy and nutrients. Anything higher than that, and you're probably adding more calories than you need.

- Supplement a frozen meal with additional veggies, dairy, and fruit to make it more well-rounded, especially if it lacks a decent amount of these foods.

- Check ingredient lists and choose one that has a shorter list and one with more recognizable ingredients.

- Choose a meal with no more than 2 grams of saturated fat and no trans fat. Take another look at the ingredient list and ensure it has no partially hydrogenated oil to ensure there is no trans fat.

- Choose a meal that contains no more than 600 mg of sodium, and look for the claims of "low sodium" or "no sodium added" on the front of the package.

- Look for meals that contain whole grains, preferably ones that have at least 5 grams or more of fiber.

10. Sugary cereal

Many of us ate them as children, and many of us probably still feed them to our children or eat them ourselves. These sugar-coated cereals are a sweet treat, but they are filled with sugar and refined grains, both of which are gut-busters. Many also lack the fiber that is so important for a healthy gut. Some cereals are made with whole grains but still have the sugary coating for better taste. Taking a walk up and down the cereal aisle can be a daunting task. Your best bet is to avoid looking at all the confusing claims on the front of the box and turn right to the nutrition facts panel. Here are a few tips to help you choose a better cereal for your gut and your health:

- Take a look at the serving size. Everything on the label, including calories, sugar, fiber, and so on, pertains to that serving size. For cereal the general serving size can be anywhere from 1/2 to 1 1/2 cups, and many people eat more than the stated serving size. If you eat double the serving size, you need to double all the nutrition facts.

- Choose a cereal that has fewer than 200 calories per serving. This allows you to add other foods to breakfast such as fruit and low-fat or fat-free dairy and still remain within a decent calorie target for the meal.

- Opt for cereals made with whole grains that nourish good gut bacteria. Look for the key first ingredients to read "100% whole." If the box merely states "whole grain," at least half of the grains in the cereal come from whole grains, but the other half is still refined grains.

- Check the fiber content and choose a cereal with at least 5 grams or more of fiber per serving. Fiber is beneficial for your gut and your health and can keep you feeling fuller longer throughout the morning.

- Choose a cereal with less than 220 mg of sodium per serving.

- Keep sugar in check and choose one with less than 10 grams per serving. Even though a cereal may be made with whole grains it can still be sky high in sugar, so check those labels.

10 Foods to Include

Just as there are foods that are known culprits for gut health there are also foods that can be helpful in protecting and keeping your gut healthy and/or reducing symptoms of GI disorders. That doesn't mean that one specific food will do the magic trick for you but adding these foods to an already healthy gut meal plan can make an even bigger impact. Keep in mind though that just because a food is generally considered healthy for your gut that doesn't mean it will be that way for everyone. Some people may be sensitive to certain foods that will then cause GI symptoms, even though these foods are gut healthy for the majority of people. Many types of foods can be potential gut helpers, but we will talk about some of the best ones.

1. Greek yogurt

Yogurt is one of the best foods to keep your gut healthy and on track. Yogurt is a cultured or fermented milk product. These products are soured and thickened by adding lactic acid–producing cultures or healthy bacteria to milk. These healthy bacteria, better known as *probiotics*, include strains such as *Lactobacillus bulgaricus*, *Streptococcus thermophilus*, *Lactobacillus acidophilus*, *Lactobacillus casei* and/or *bifidus*. All of these probiotics in yogurts have the ability to help maintain the correct balance of "good" to "bad" bacteria by replenishing the normal gut flora within the GI tract that is needed to boost immunity and promote a healthy digestive system. Greek yogurt is even better than regular yogurt because it contains probiotics and a higher protein content. When choosing a yogurt, take a look at calorie, fat, and sugar content as well as calcium, especially if you use yogurt as a significant source of calcium in your diet. Choosing a non-fat or low-fat version with live and active cultures, vitamin D, and at least 200 mg of calcium per serving is a healthy choice. As far as sugar content goes, keep in mind that this will include both added sugar and the naturally occurring sugar from milk and fruit, if it is included. Choose a yogurt with less than 15 grams of sugar per serving, and stay away from yogurts that include high-fructose corn syrup in the ingredient list. Beware of yogurts with artificial sweeteners, as they often contain sugar alcohols, which for some people can cause GI symptoms. Soy yogurt is a good alternative for those who are vegetarians or lactose intolerant (though, interestingly, many people with lactose intolerance can tolerate yogurt without a problem). Soy yogurt is similar to yogurt made from dairy in terms of calories, protein, and probiotics. Frozen yogurt can work, though you need to check the package specifically to see whether it has live and active cultures. The freezing process won't kill the live and active cultures, but not all frozen yogurt products contain them. Yogurt makes a great breakfast, lunch, or snack. You can jazz it up with ground flaxseed, low-fat granola, and fresh fruit or even use it to whip up a smoothie.

Your Nutrition Solution Tidbit: Not all yogurts and yogurt products are the same. Always look for the words "live and active cultures" on the label to ensure it contains the probiotics you expect. If you see anything else, such as "live cultures" or "active cultures," the product probably does not have the probiotics you are looking for. Check all the yogurts within a brand, as some flavors within a same brand name can differ in this regard.

2. Oatmeal

Start your day with fiber-rich oatmeal instead of a sugary breakfast cereal or a piece of white bread, both of which will do your gut no good at all. Whole oats are filling, low in fat, chock full of soluble fiber, and rich in nutrients such as selenium, thiamin, phosphorus, and manganese. Oatmeal is beneficial for your entire digestive tract, especially your colon because of its high content of soluble fibers. For those who suffer from IBD (Crohn's disease or ulcerative colitis), oatmeal can be especially helpful during non–flare-up times. Steel-cut oats contain an even higher nutrient content than rolled or quick oats. You can go a step further and add fresh fruit, a pinch of cinnamon, nuts, and/or raisins to boost the nutrition content and taste even more.

3. Ground flaxseed

Some call it one of the most powerful plant foods on the planet. Flaxseed can add tremendous benefits to your gut health. It acts as an anti-inflammatory and is rich in omega-3 fatty acids, particularly in the form *linolenic acid* (ALA). It also contains plenty of soluble fiber and natural oils to help the digestive process along and promote regularity, as well as vitamins, minerals, and *lignans*, which contain antioxidants and plant estrogens. Ground flaxseed is much better absorbed than its whole counterpart, which basically passes through your system without being digested. You can add about 1 to 2 tablespoons of ground flaxseed per day to your meal plan, but you probably shouldn't use more than that. Flaxseed is usually not recommended during pregnancy. Add ground flaxseed to smoothies, non-fat yogurt, hot cereal, mashed potatoes, or in baked goods. Start small and increase slowly to avoid gastric upset.

4. Cranberries

Cranberries aren't just for Thanksgiving anymore. One of the best-known uses for cranberries as a functional food is for the prevention and treatment of urinary tract infections (UTIs). Out of all the fruits and vegetables out there, cranberries contain one of the highest levels of antioxidants and phytonutrients. Cranberries help support the cardiovascular and immune systems, help decrease the risk of tooth and gum diseases, and play a role in digestive tract support, as well. They help decrease adherence of *H. pylori* to the walls of the stomach and suppress its growth, thus decreasing the risk of gastric ulcers. In addition, the antioxidant and anti-inflammatory properties help decrease the risk of colon cancer. Researchers are also finding that this small but powerful fruit may help to optimize the balance of good and bad bacteria in our gut, making it more favorable to good digestive health. Cranberries are available fresh, frozen, dried, or in juice form. Be aware that drinking too much cranberry juice can cause mild side effects in some people such as stomach upset and diarrhea. Drinking large quantities (more an one liter per day) for long periods of time may also increase the risk of kidney stones. Precautions should be taken by those who are pregnant, have an allergy to aspirin, gastritis, diabetes, low stomach acid, or kidney stones, or who are taking warfarin and other medications.

Your Nutrition Solution Tidbit: When choosing cranberry juice, look for 100-percent fruit juice. Avoid those that are packaged as "drinks" or "cocktails," which means they contain loads of sugar and very little actual cranberry juice. If choosing sweetened cranberry juice, choose a brand with the least amount of sugar. Don't forget that sugar can damage the healthy bacteria that you are trying to increase. Cranberry juice is often mixed with other juices to increase its palatability. For the best health benefits, however, consider using an unsweetened cranberry juice that has no added sugar and is not mixed with other juices and not made from a concentrate. You can try diluting the juice with water or adding a few drops of stevia to cut the tartness.

5. Kefir

Kefir is a fermented dairy food that is similar to a drinkable yogurt. Fermented foods are full of probiotics. Kefir is easily digested and one of the most probiotic-rich foods you can find. Like yogurt, kefir contains live and active cultures. Kefir also contains *oligosaccharides* (a type of prebiotic) and complex carbohydrates that act as food to the beneficial bacteria in the gut. Keeping these bacteria happy and fed with a highly nutritional food such as kefir will supercharge your immune system and help create a healthier digestive system. Kefir's superior nutritional content includes vitamin B12, calcium, magnesium, folate, biotin, and enzymes. In addition to boosting the immune system and supporting digestive health, kefir can also help heal IBD and IBS, build bone density, battle allergies, improve lactose intolerance, kill *candida* (a strain of yeast that causes fungal infections), fight cancer, and support detoxification. Regular use of kefir can help relieve all types of intestinal disorders and symptoms as well as promote regular bowel movements, reduce gas, and create a good balance of "good" and "bad" bacteria in your gut. Choose a brand with a lower sugar content, and be sure to keep it cold, as the cultures can easily be destroyed by heat.

Your Nutrition Solution Tidbit: In addition to yogurt and kefir, other probiotic-rich fermented foods include sauerkraut, kimchi, and tempeh.

6. Asparagus

As a prebiotic, asparagus has tremendous benefits for your gut. Asparagus is rich in *fructooligosaccharides* (FOS), a type of soluble fiber, and *inulin*, a short-chain fructan. Both have been shown to be power foods for probiotics. This vegetable also helps to increase the absorption of minerals such as calcium, can reduce the risk of colon cancer by keeping things moving through your GI tract, and acts as an anti-inflammatory. Asparagus contains plenty of antioxidants and other nutrients such as vitamin K, folate, copper, B vitamins, potassium, zinc, vitamin A, and even a bit of protein. Asparagus can be enjoyed in many ways, but to get the full benefits and retain the most nutrients, stick with fresh, washed asparagus that has been steamed, microwaved, roasted, or sautéed. Don't overcook.

7. Bananas

What a great fruit! Bananas are easy to eat, easy to digest, are a sweet treat, and can benefit the entire digestive system. Bananas offer specific benefits for those who suffer from GI symptoms such as constipation, diarrhea, and an upset stomach. This bright yellow fruit is a rich source of FOS, one of the prebiotics I discussed earlier. When probiotics or beneficial bacteria are well-fed with prebiotics such as those in bananas, those good bacteria can establish a strong presence in the gut to help fend off overgrowth of pathogenic organisms such as yeast. Probiotics don't stand a chance if there are no prebiotics in the gut to help nourish them. Bananas are chock full of all types of essential nutrients, too, including potassium, vitamin C, vitamin B6, manganese, and fiber. Because of their high levels of magnesium and potassium, bananas are known to reduce inflammation and support heart health. You can enjoy bananas in many different ways: by themselves, sliced on oatmeal or a whole-grain cereal, in yogurt, or even smothered with peanut butter. Make sure you eat bananas at the right time: if they are underripe, they have a higher acid content, which for some can cause digestive issues. So make sure they are not too green on the outside.

8. Jerusalem artichoke

A Jerusalem artichoke is actually a species of sunflower. The part we are interested in is a *tuber*, or root vegetable, that acts as a potent prebiotic for your digestive system. It is different than the globe artichoke, a type of edible flower bud that you're probably used to seeing in grocery stores. It is eaten much the same way as a potato. Jerusalem artichokes are an excellent source of fiber and are especially high in oligofructose inulin, a prebiotic. These tubers contain both soluble and insoluble fiber, which help reduce constipation and protect against colon cancer. It also contains some B vitamins and antioxidants, such as vitamin C, A, and E, as well as flavonoid compounds, such as carotenes, that help offer protection from certain cancers, inflammation, and age-related diseases. They are also a good source of minerals and electrolytes, especially potassium, iron, and copper, helping this vegetable to be heart health friendly. Jerusalem artichokes are very versatile and can be cooked in many different ways. They can be enjoyed raw in salads or boiled, mashed, roasted, or sautéed as you would a potato. Be careful not to overcook them as they can turn soft and mushy quickly.

9. Black beans

Any legume (dried beans and lentils) will help to release short-chain fatty acids (SCFA) that help to strengthen intestinal cells and improve the absorption of vitamins and minerals (micronutrients). The American Diabetes Association, the American Heart Association, the American Cancer Society, and the Dietary Guidelines for Americans all recommend legumes/dried beans as a key food for the prevention of disease and for optimizing health. Beans contain prebiotics, which feed the "good" bacteria to help them thrive. The starch in beans is *resistant starch*, meaning that the starch stays intact until it reaches the large intestine, where it nourishes the "good" bacteria. Increasing your consumption of legumes can help decrease the risk for colon cancer. Black beans in particular provide special support for gut health, especially for the colon. Black beans contain more resistant starch than most other beans and legumes. They seem to contain the perfect mix of substances to allow the bacteria in the colon to produce *butyric acid*, which is essential for the health and proper functioning of the colon. All legumes are packed with fiber, protein, folate, B vitamins, and other essential nutrients, all of which play a role in regulating gut health. Black beans take it even further: the color of the bean comes from *anthocyanins*, flavonoid pigments that offer extraordinary antioxidant and anti-inflammatory benefits. Black beans also have a low glycemic index (GI), meaning that the sugar they contain is absorbed slowly into the bloodstream, which helps keep blood sugar levels steady. This can help greatly with blood sugar issues as well as helping to prevent food cravings, which in turn can help with weight loss. Low GI foods such as black beans can help to fight the insulin resistance that is associated with diabetes and lower the risk of heart disease and stroke. You can find legumes dried or canned all year long. Although legumes are extremely healthy foods, many people tend to avoid them because they are known for causing gas. If this is a problem for you, try soaking them in water with a small amount of baking soda or vinegar before cooking; and be sure to change the water and rinse them thoroughly before cooking. Cook them slowly to help decrease the gas-causing compounds. If you don't want to deal with that you can also purchase canned beans, but make sure to rinse them thoroughly before cooking. Eat beans in small amounts and eat them with other foods to help decrease gas production. Beans are so versatile and inexpensive. You can add them to soups, casseroles, stews, salads, chili, whole-grain pasta dishes, brown rice, Mexican dishes, and dips, just to name a few.

10. Blueberries

All berries have a balanced glucose-to-fructose ratio, which makes them easier on the gut than fruits that have a higher fructose content. Blueberries are considered one of the "superfoods." They have the highest antioxidant content among all fruits and vegetables. The pigment that gives them their bold, blue color is also a powerful antioxidant called anthocyanin, the same flavonoid found in black beans. Blueberries contain a whole host of other phytonutrients that possess both antioxidant and anti-inflammatory properties and that have a very positive impact on gut health and normal bowel function. Blueberries have been found to strengthen memory, improve immune function, provide cardiovascular benefits, stabilize blood sugar, improve eye health, prevent certain cancers, and diversify gut bacteria. Blueberries are high in vitamin K, manganese, vitamin C, copper, and fiber. They also contain polysaccharide prebiotics that feed and nourish good bacteria. The nutrients in blueberries, along with its fructose content, improve digestion by stimulating the gastric and digestive juices to move food smoothly and properly through your digestive tract. You can use blueberries as a healthy snack by themselves, added on top of your oatmeal or whole-grain cereal, mixed into yogurt, or added to a salad. Keep in mind that all berries are gut-friendly foods, so enjoy your blackberries, strawberries, raspberries, and cranberries, as well.

Gut-Friendly Herbs and Spices

Some of the most common herbs and spices that we use in cooking on a daily basis may just be beneficial for the digestive system.

Ginger

Herbalists have recommended the root of the ginger plant for thousands of years to help relieve gastrointestinal issues. Ginger can help protect against colon cancer, boost the immune system, and act as an anti-inflammatory. You can try grating ginger in a dressing of extra virgin olive oil, lemon juice, minced garlic, and a little sea salt to top vegetables and salads. This mixture, along with a little orange juice, can make a great marinade for fish and meat. Grated ginger goes well with stir-fries and meat dishes and is tasty in homemade baked goods as well as made into a tea. There are plenty of ways to include and enjoy ginger in your diet. Powdered capsule supplements are also available, but it is important to keep in mind that the supplement can act as a blood thinner, so let your doctor know if you plan to take this or any other herb in supplement form.

Coriander

Coriander is a spice whose seeds contain powerful, cell-protecting antioxidants. This spice is said to help soothe digestive ailments and support digestion. It may soothe symptoms of IBS and other gut disorders by relaxing the contracted or spastic digestive muscles that cause the discomfort. Although coriander is sold in a powdered form, it is best to use the whole seeds, as the beneficial oil tends to dissipate after a few months once it is ground. You can use coriander as a tea by boiling one teaspoon of coriander seeds in one cup of water, steeping for five to ten minutes, then straining and enjoying. You can use coriander seeds in chili, soups, stews, or casseroles, or grind the seeds and use on meat or fish as a dry rub before cooking.

Fennel

Dried fennel seeds come from a plant in the celery family. It is popular in Italian and Mediterranean dishes, and has been used as a digestive aid all over the world. The seeds contain a large amount of *anethole*, a compound also found in anise, which helps with various digestive problems including IBS, heartburn, intestinal gas, indigestion, and bloating. Fennel has anti-spastic properties and helps stimulate the production of gastric juices for more efficient digestion. Fennel can be used in lentil dishes, with potatoes, in stew and sauces, and works well with cinnamon.

Cumin

Cumin is on top of the list of herbs and spices that support healthy digestion. The flavorful seeds are an excellent source of iron, and have been shown to stimulate the production of pancreatic enzymes, which are necessary for proper digestion. These seeds promote healthy absorption of nutrients, as well. You can purchase cumin as whole seeds or in powder form, though the seeds keep their flavor longer. Add cumin to lentils, beans, brown rice, and sautéed vegetables. You can even use the seeds to make tea.

Cayenne pepper

Most people with digestive issues shy away from cayenne pepper because of its spiciness. However, cayenne is actually a digestive *soother*. Cayenne stimulates the digestive process by promoting healthy muscle movement throughout the GI tract, and helps stimulate the production of digestive acids, which aid in the proper breakdown and absorption of nutrients. If that weren't enough, cayenne may even help repair a damaged gut, including stomach ulcers and damage to the intestinal lining. One 2006 study in *Critical Reviews in Food Science and Nutrition* found that capsaicin, the primary compound found in the pepper that makes it hot, actually helps to stimulate the secretions and gastric mucosal blood flow that aid in the healing of stomach ulcers. (Source: Satyanarayana, M.N. "Capsaicin and Gastric Ulcers." *Critical Reviews in Food Science and Nutrition*, 46.4 (2006): 275–328. National Center for Biotechnology Information, U.S. National Library of Medicine/PubMed.gov. Webpage accessed January 28, 2015.) This spice acts an anti-inflammatory and immune booster, as well. You can use cayenne pepper fresh or as a dried powder. It goes well in just about any type of dish—even chocolate!

chapter 5

menu planning and shopping guide

Now that you have learned the most effective ways to increase your gut health, it is time to put that information to work for you by organizing your weekly menus and grocery lists. Eating for a healthy gut is all about eating a healthy and clean diet—the type of eating plan that will not only be beneficial for your gut but for your overall health, as well. Remember that this needs to be a permanent change. This chapter will provide helpful tips to get started on the right foods with your new and improved way of eating. Properly navigating the grocery store, menu planning, and mastering food labels will be key tools in your arsenal that will help you choose foods that will improve gut health and help treat symptoms you may be dealing with. It is worth stating again that if you know you are intolerant of or sensitive to any food(s), be sure to avoid it/them.

Menu Planning Tips

Controlling symptoms of digestive disorders and promoting a healthier gut requires paying close attention to the foods that you purchase, prepare, and consume. Eating healthier and cleaner, shooting for a healthy weight, engaging in regular exercise, and managing daily stress are just some of the lifestyle changes that will have a big impact on your gut health. We have discussed all of these previously, but here are a few more tips to help you easily plan daily menus and be prepared for special circumstances:

Get the whole family on board. It will be easier to plan menus if others in your household are on board with this new healthier way of eating. The best part is that it will benefit the entire family. Don't make the mistake of preparing one dish for yourself and another for the family. Explain to them the changes you will be making for your health and for theirs, and why it is important. The more informed they are, and the better they understand why changes are being made, the easier it will be for them to accept these changes. This is the perfect time to teach kids good dietary habits they will keep for a lifetime.

Plan ahead. Write out menus for the week so you are able to plan meals that avoid foods you shouldn't have and include the ones you should. Cook meals at home and bring lunches to work or school until you get a better handle on your new eating style. The more prepared you are, the less likely you will be to eat out, eat on the run, or grab something you shouldn't—all of which can spell trouble and sabotage your best intentions. Once your weekly menus are planned, it's time to create a shopping list. This will help you buy only what is on the list and not stray to foods that should be avoided.

Don't change your entire diet all at once. Take small steps to begin making changes. Start with breakfast, then move on to snacks, and so on. Each time you make a change, stick with it until it becomes permanent; then, move on to another. Trying to change your entire diet all at once can be overwhelming and can lead to failure, even with the best of intentions.

Look for new recipes to incorporate into your meal plan that include gut-healthy foods. There are tons of fresh, healthy foods that fit into this type of eating style to explore and experience; the easiest way to do this is to try new recipes. Look for recipes that are gut-healthy, anti-inflammatory, Mediterranean style, or clean eating. All of these will help you stick to a healthy gut way of life.

When planning meals and snacks, incorporate the foods that I listed in Chapter 4, including those spices and herbs. Choose a variety of foods, espcially of fruits and vegetables, to get the full range of essential vitamin, minerals, antioxidants, and phytonutrients. Keep this book and other resources handy while meal planning, so that you can go back and visit them when you have questions or even need a little motivation.

Be prepared for meals and snacks away from home. Don't put yourself in the situation of having to hit the drive-thru.

Include a few meatless meals in your weekly meal plan. You will find them just as satisfying and may just find a few new favorites.

Avoid your personal trigger foods. Don't assume that because a certain fruit or vegetable, for example, causes digestive issues, you are intolerant or sensitive to *all* fruits and vegetables. Keep a food diary so that you know which specific foods you need to stay away from; do not avoid whole food groups. A food diary is a good tool to help you create an eating plan that will make you and your gut happy.

Be creative with substitutions for the foods that trigger you so that you don't feel you are being deprived.

Your Nutrition Solution Tidbit: If sitting down and writing out weekly menu and shopping lists is not appealing to you or seems like a daunting task than grab your phone and find an app for that! There are plenty of apps out there for smartphones that can make meal planning and shopping lists easy and fun.

Don't forget snacks

Believe it or not snacks are an important part of your meal plan. Eating five or six small meals a day is a great way to eat, for so many reasons. It gives you more opportunities to get in all of the servings of the healthy food groups you need daily; it keeps meals smaller so you don't feel overstuffed, bloated, and uncomfortable; it keeps blood sugar levels stable and, thus, your appetite an even keel; it keeps you in control for your next meal; and it sustains energy levels throughout the day. Keep your snacks healthy, watch portion sizes, and don't forget to add snacks to menu plans and grocery lists. Here are a few snack ideas to get you started:

- Celery sticks with hummus
- Almonds and raisins
- Apple slices with nutbutter
- Zucchini sticks with salsa
- Fresh grapes and walnuts
- Raw cauliflower with bean dip
- Plain popcorn
- Fresh berries
- Whole-grain cereal, fat-free almond milk, and sliced banana
- Smoothie made with frozen fruit, soy milk, and ground flaxseed
- Greek yogurt topped with low-fat granola
- Fresh avocado and carrots

Swap it out

When you change your diet for better health, it can sometimes feel as though you're giving up everything you love to eat. It can be hard to give up the favorite foods that you are used to eating and enjoying. The good news is that there is no need to feel deprived if you learn to make some smart and simple swaps that can reduce calories, sugar, and unhealthy fat as well as help you avoid any foods that trigger digestive issues for you. These swap ideas will help get you started. As you get used to your new eating approach, you will surely master the art of swapping!

Instead of:	Try:
Wheat flours/grains*	Arrowroot, buckwheat, millet, quinoa, rice, potato starch, soy, tapioca, corn, wheat-free pasta, couscous, beans, potatoes
Table sugar	Honey, pure maple syrup, fruit puree
Salad dressing	Extra-virgin olive oil with vinegar, lemon juice, and a little ginger
Mayonnaise	Pureed avocado or homemade guacamole
Milk	Lactose-free milk, almond or rice milk, soy milk

Ice Cream	Frozen bananas and berries, blended or low-fat frozen yogurt
Milkshake	Smoothie made with soy/almond milk, ground flaxseed, and frozen fruit(s)
Soft drinks/soda	Green tea over ice, sweetened with a little honey and lemon
Apple pie	Fresh apple sprinkled with cinnamon and baked
Fast food French fries	Freshly cut potato (white or sweet potato), drizzled with olive oil and oven-baked
Potato chips and dip	Homemade guacamole and raw veggies
Pizza	Homemade whole-wheat pita bread, pizza sauce (watch the sugar content), part-skim mozzarella cheese, and vegetables
Burgers	Turkey burger (ground lean turkey breast) or a portabella mushroom brushed with extra-virgin olive oil and grilled; try a lettuce wrap instead of a bun or use a thin whole-grain sandwich bagel, add lettuce, tomato, onion, and other favorite veggie toppings

You only need to substitute for wheat if you have an allergy, intolerance, or sensitivity. The suggestions in the previous table are only a few examples of the kinds of things you can safely substitute for wheat. If you cannot eat wheat, visit with an RDN who can teach you all you need to know about avoiding wheat completely. To correctly substitute for any food, of course, always read labels and ingredient lists.

Whatever it is you like to eat, you can find a substitute that will be healthier and easier on your gut. It may take a little time to figure it out, but eventually you will be swapping out foods like a champ and enjoying it!

Navigating the Supermarket

Consuming a diet that will promote a healthier gut starts well before you sit down to eat. You need to be armed with a well-thought-out weekly meal plan and grocery list. Even with all of that in your arsenal, navigating your way through aisles and aisles of food—and temptations—can be overwhelming. Leave yourself plenty of time to grocery shop so that you are able to shop wisely and knowledgeably. The goal is to stock your kitchen with healthy, wholesome foods that will fit perfectly into your new eating style. Keep a running list of foods and beverages you need throughout the week, so that when you go to the grocery store you can stock up. Stocking your kitchen with gut-healthy foods will make it easier to stick to your goals. It may take more time at first, but as you master the knowledge of which foods are better than others, grocery shopping will be a snap. Always get in a healthy meal or snack before you go shopping: Visiting the grocery store on an empty stomach can be your worst enemy!

Many of the larger chains allow you to create an online shopping list, and offer guidelines and meal ideas for specific health conditions. In addition, many of these stores now employ registered dietitians on the premises, so if you get stuck or have questions, don't be afraid to ask! Take advantage of the nutritional and cooking classes that many offer, too.

Grocery stores can be challenging, with all of those foods you should avoid, staring you in the face at every turn. Your number-one weapon will be a well-organized grocery list that follows your pre-planned menu for the week. It will help make grocery shopping more bearable and even enjoyable.

Produce section

The first section to greet you in most grocery stores is the produce section that is full of all types of fresh fruits and vegetables in a rainbow of colors. This will be the largest section of the grocery store and the one you should spend most of your time in. Fruits and vegetables are chock full of nutrients, phytochemicals, and the probiotics and prebiotics that are promoters of a healthy gut. These foods make healthy, low-calorie snacks and should be included with every meal. Fruit can be a great substitution for sugary desserts if you have a sweet tooth. With the many types of fruits and vegetables available, if you don't like one, there is surely another one out there that you will. A few tips on shopping this section:

- Look for produce with the deepest color. The more colorful the produce, the more nutrients and phytochemicals it contains. But keep in mind that even white veggies such as onions and cauliflower contain loads of beneficial nutrients, too. In fact, onions contain a phytochemical called *quercetin* that has anti-inflammatory and immune- boosting properties and can help lower the risk of cancer, heart disease, and type 2 diabetes.

- Choose a variety of fruits and vegetables. Variety is the spice of life, and the greater variety you choose, the more nutritional value you will get in return. Be adventurous and try something new every week. You never know what you might find that you really like.

- Buy fresh fruits and vegetables that are in season. You can always buy frozen when they are not in season. Opt for locally grown produce and organic when possible. The fresher they are the more nutritional value they have.

- Pre-cut fruits and vegetables can be convenient for the busy person and family on the go. They are also more expensive, so consider cutting them up yourself and placing them in airtight containers so they are always available in the fridge.

- When picking fruits and vegetables look them over thoroughly and choose the freshest ones that are free from bruises, soft spots, or gashes.

- When buying canned fruit, choose varieties that are canned in 100-percent juice and have no syrup added, which can add loads of refined sugar.

- When buying canned vegetables, choose ones that are labeled "no salt" or "low sodium." Regular canned foods can be high in sodium.

- Buy only what you need so that you can eat it before it begins to spoil and lose its nutritional value.

- Nuts and seeds are often found in this section and should be a regular part of your grocery list. They can add healthy fat, fiber, and other nutritional value to your meals to help maintain good digestive health.

Dairy section

The dairy section can be found on the perimeter of the grocery store. Even though it is usually labeled the "dairy case," it doesn't just contain dairy. In addition to foods such as milk, you'll also find milk alternatives such as soymilk; yogurts; cheeses; sour cream; cream cheese; eggs; pudding; butter and margarine; and hummus and other dips and spreads.

Choose low-fat and fat-free versions of everything to lower your intake of unhealthy saturated fats.

Check labels on margarines and spreads for the words "partially hydrogenated" in the list of ingredients. These are the unhealthy trans fats and should be avoided at all costs. Many varieties of margarine are now made without trans fats. Better yet, ditch the margarine and butter and choose olive oil or a nut butter instead.

Choose yogurt that is fat-free, low-fat, or "light/lite." Greek yogurt is a great option because it provides more protein than regular yogurt. To get the full probiotic benefits of yogurt, check the packaging and make sure it states "live and active cultures."

Although eggs are considered a protein source, you can find eggs, egg whites, and egg substitutes in this section, as well. Egg whites and egg substitutes are great alternatives for whole eggs and a great way to lower your fat and cholesterol intake.

If you are lactose intolerant, or if dairy foods tend to cause digestive symptoms for you, swap these foods for others that provide the same type of nutrients so you won't miss out. You can swap regular milk for soy milk, almond milk, or rice milk to avoid lactose. You can also try soy yogurt and/or soy cheese in place of their regular dairy counterparts. Check labels to ensure these foods are fortified with calcium and vitamin D because we tend to get these nutrients mostly from milk products. Interestingly, many people who are lactose intolerant can tolerate yogurt, so don't rule out all dairy if milk is a problem. You may need to experiment a bit to see what dairy foods you can tolerate and in what amounts.

Meat and seafood section

The meat and seafood section (sometimes two separate areas) is yet another area that can be found in the perimeter of the grocery store. This section includes fresh meats, seafood, and fish as well as the deli section. Meats, especially red meats, can contain high amounts of unhealthy saturated fats, cholesterol, and other gut-busters. The goal in this section is to choose leaner meats and fish to help lower your risk for health and heart issues and promote a healthier gut.

Choose lean meats such as skinless white meat poultry, fish (wild caught), pork loin, pork tenderloin, or ground turkey or chicken breast. Choose red meat only occasionally, and only the leanest cuts, including top sirloin steak, eye of round roast or steak, top round roast and steak, flank steak, and extra-lean ground beef (at least 90 percent or more lean). A cut of meat is considered lean if it includes the words "round" or "loin."

Opt for grass-fed beef as opposed to grain fed. Grass-fed beef contains omega-3 fatty acids, giving it a healthier ratio of omega 6 to omega 3 fats; contains slightly less saturated fat and twice as much CLA (*conjugated linoleic acid*, a fatty acid that is associated with some beneficial health effects) as grain-fed beef.

When it comes to deli meat, choose lean turkey, roast beef, lean ham, or chicken breast and stay away from meats that are full of saturated fat such as bologna and salami. Keep an eye on sodium content and choose nitrate-free meat whenever possible.

Eat fish as often as possible, especially fatty fish that contains healthy omega-3 fatty acids: salmon, tuna, trout, herring, sardines, and mackerel.

Your Nutrition Solution Tidbit: The American Heart Association recommends that people consume at least two servings of fish per week.

Bread, cereal, rice, and pasta aisles

As you get into the center aisles of the grocery store, you will encounter fewer fresh foods and more packaged and processed foods such as canned goods, bread, cereal, rice, and pasta. These foods are great ways to get your daily whole-grain and fiber intake as well as other essential nutrients, *if* you make the right choices. Making the wrong choices can lead to an unhealthy gut and the very digestive symptoms that you are trying to avoid. Here's how to navigate these aisles with aplomb:

- Avoid refined foods such as white bread, regular pasta, white rice, and sugary cereal, and choose the whole-wheat or whole-grain versions instead. Take a look back at Chapter 3 for more tips on choosing whole grains.

- Choose oatmeal, a hearty whole grain that is high in fiber. Steel-cut oats are a great choice. Regular oatmeal is better than instant because it is less processed, but even instant oatmeal is a whole grain and hence an improvement over sugary cereal. Watch the sugar content of flavored instant oatmeal. Flavor it yourself with cinnamon, honey, pure maple syrup, raisins, and other fruits.

- When choosing dry cereals, choose varieties that state "whole grain" on the label, and aim for at least 5 grams of fiber or more per serving. Read the label for sugar content as well and stick to ones that contain less than 10 grams of sugar per serving.

- Opt for whole-grain foods such as brown or wild rice as opposed to white rice. Choose plain rice over pre-packaged, flavored rice, which is more processed and usually contains tons of sodium.

- Try alternate whole grains such as bulgur, quinoa, barley, and whole-grain couscous for something different.

- Reading the food labels is key in all sections but especially in these. Read labels and ingredient lists to ensure you are choosing foods that are truly made of whole grains and have the fiber content you expect without all of the refined sugar and sodium.

Canned food aisle

The canned food section includes foods such as fruits, vegetables, tuna and salmon, beans, soup, bullion, and more. Keeping a variety of healthier canned goods on hand can ensure you always have something to reach for in a pinch. Though not fresh, they can still add plenty of nutrients to your required daily servings of certain foods groups. Canned foods can be nutritious if you make the right choices:

- Choose fruit that is canned in water or its own natural juices to keep sugar content down. Stay away from ones in syrup.
- Choose vegetables that state "no salt" or "low (or no) sodium."
- Avoid buying canned vegetables that contain added fat and sodium. No need to ruin a good thing!
- Choose tuna or salmon that is packed in water as opposed to packed in oils.
- Choose lower fat and lower sodium soups and stick with the broth-based soups that contain loads of vegetables. You can always add more veggies of your own too!
- Try beans such as black beans, kidney, lentils, garbanzos, and navy beans with no added salt, to add

to soups, casseroles, whole-wheat pasta dishes, and salads as an extra protein, nutrient, and fiber boost. Rinse canned beans to remove as much sodium as possible. Bean dishes make a great alternative to meat dishes.

Oils, condiments, and dressings aisle

This can be a dangerous section of the store because it is filled with foods that contain plenty of fat, sodium, sugar, and calories. Making the right choices in this aisle is essential to a healthier gut.

Choose healthier oils such as extra-virgin olive oil and canola oil and use them sparingly. A small amount can go a long way and can pack in a lot of calories. Use them in place of unhealthier fats to get the full benefit.

Keep in mind that ketchup, salsa, and other condiments can contain loads of sodium and refined sugar. Choose lower sugar and sodium versions, or choose brands with the lowest amount of sugar and sodium per serving.

Choose salad dressings that are oil-based, not cream-based, and are labeled as "reduced fat" or "light." Compare labels to choose brands that are lower in calories, fat, sodium, and sugar. Your best choice for salad dressing is a drizzle of extra virgin olive oil with vinegar or a little lemon or lime juice.

Replace regular, full-fat mayonnaise with a reduced-fat or fat-free version; better yet, substitute pureed avocado, guacamole, or hummus for something more nutritious.

Your Nutrition Solution Tidbit: When you're buying oil, always opt for extra-virgin olive oil (EVOO)—the purest form of olive oil and the oil with the lowest acidity. EVOO is great for dressings, drizzling on veggies, or brushing on breads. If you plan to cook with it, it's best to go with virgin or light/lite olive oil, as both are better suited for heating. Always check dates, because oils have a limited shelf life; grab a bottle from the back of the shelf, as light tends to destroy the oil and its properties. Store it in a dark, cool, dry place once you get home.

Frozen foods section

The frozen food section includes frozen vegetables, fruits, pizza, entrées, breakfast foods, specialty items, breads, juices, desserts, and the list goes on. Frozen fruits and vegetables can be a convenient way to keep produce on hand, especially during the winter months. Frozen produce is flash frozen at the peak of its freshness and is just as good as fresh in terms of nutritional content. Frozen foods can be convenient when you don't have time to cook, but just as you do in the other sections of the grocery store, you need to make the right choices:

- Always read food labels in the freezer section. There are a wide variety of foods and you can always choose healthier varieties. Quick example: If you are buying waffles, opt for a whole-grain version.

- Choose vegetables without sauces and butters. Many frozen vegetables come in ready-to-steam bags, which makes it even more convenient to add vegetables to soups, casseroles, pasta dishes, and stews, or just have them as a side dish.

- Choose frozen fruit without added sugar. Frozen fruits are great for making smoothies or for adding to whole-grain waffles for breakfast or to yogurt as a snack. Choose organic when possible.

- When choosing frozen meals/entrées, always read the nutrition facts panel first. These meals are fine on occasion when you don't have time to cook, but don't rely on them regularly. Refer to Chapter 4 on general guidelines for frozen entrées. Never assume these meals are healthy without first checking the labels.

Using Food Labels for a Healthier Gut

To truly follow a healthier approach to eating, you need to become a food label reader so that you can determine, without guessing, whether a food is healthy and whether it will fit into your gut-healthy meal plan. The food label is regulated by the FDA and is full of great information, including the nutrition facts panel, nutrient content claims, health claims, and allergen information. Food labels are meant to be used by the consumer to compare foods and make better choices. They are helpful whether you are trying to follow a specific diet, trying to avoid foods/ingredients you may be sensitive or allergic to, or just trying to eat healthier.

The nutrition facts panel

The nutrition facts panel provides consumers with information about the nutrients that we should be most concerned with. This panel is the rectangular box on the back or side of a packaged food or beverage that contains all of the pertinent nutritional information. The nutrition facts panel was mandated under the Nutrition Labeling and Education Act (NLEA) of 1990 and is based on recommendations from the Food and Drug Administration (FDA) and the U.S. Department of Agriculture (USDA). The panel can help you manage your gut health, your overall health, and your weight.

You can use the nutrition facts panel to your advantage by following a few simple tips:

Size it up

One of the first parts of the label is the serving size, which is usually expressed in weight, volume, or number of units. Take a close look at the serving size and the servings per container, then make a mental note of the following:

- The number of calories in a single serving.
- The number of calories in the entire package.
- The number of servings you plan to eat.

All of the nutrition information on the panel pertains to that one, specified, single serving size. Simply looking at the nutrition information won't mean much if you don't pay attention to the serving size and how many servings you plan on eating. For example, if you plan on eating

Nutrition Facts

Serving Size 1 cup (228g)
Servings Per Container about 2

Amount Per Serving

Calories 250	Calories from Fat 110

	% Daily Value*
Total Fat 12g	**18%**
Saturated Fat 3g	**15%**
Trans Fat 3g	
Cholesterol 30mg	**10%**
Sodium 470mg	**20%**
Total Carbohydrate 31g	**10%**
Dietary Fiber 0g	**0%**
Sugars 5g	
Proteins 5g	

Vitamin A	4%
Vitamin C	2%
Calcium	20%
Iron	4%

*Percent Daily Values are based on a 2,000 calorie diet. Your Daily Values may be higher or lower depending on your calorie needs.

	Calories:	2,000	2,500
Total Fat	Less than	65g	80g
Saturated Fat	Less than	20g	25g
Cholesterol	Less than	300mg	300mg
Sodium	Less than	2,400mg	2,400mg
Total Carbohydrate		300g	375g
Dietary Fiber		25g	30g

For educational purposes only. This label does not meet the labeling requirements described in 21 CFR 101.9.

two servings, you'll need to double all of the information, including calories, nutrients (such as fat), and %DV (percent daily value). When you're comparing calories and nutrients between two brands of the same food, check to see if the serving size is the same before making your comparison.

Your Nutrition Solution Tidbit: Many food packages, including beverages, contain more than one serving. Don't fall into the trap of assuming there is only one serving in a package and consuming the whole package before you read the label first. That can add up to a lot more calories, sugar, and fat then you bargained for.

Focus on calories

Next on the label are calories and, more specifically, calories from fat. This is important for determining whether a food is appropriate for your plan, especially if you are trying to lose weight. Foods that are high in calories or have many calories coming from fat can lead to weight gain. Keep the following in mind when evaluating calorie content:

- Just because a food is fat free does not mean it is calorie free or sugar free! Foods without fat are often high in refined sugar and still contain calories.

- Check to see how many total calories the food contains and how many of those calories come from fat. For example, if a food has 300 calories per serving, and 150 of those calories come from fat, then half of the calories in a single serving come from a fat source. That gives you good reason to check just what type of fat.

- If you are looking to manage your weight or lose weight, consider how the calories per serving will fit into your total calorie goal for the day. If you eat and drink more calories than you burn, you will gain weight, and, in turn, you will increase your risk for an unhealthy gut.

In general, you can use the following guide to gauge the calories in a single product (based on a 2,000-calorie diet). What really matters, though, is the total calories you consume in a day and not a single food:

Low in calories = 40 calories per serving
Moderate in calories = 100 calories per serving
High in calories = 400 calories or more per serving

Limit certain nutrients

The nutrients listed first on the label are the ones that most Americans generally consume enough or too much of in their daily diet. Nutrients to limit for better health and to promote a healthier gut include total fat, saturated fat, trans fat, cholesterol, and sodium. The goal is to stay well below the 100% daily value for each of these for the entire day. (More on daily value in a moment.) You should know how much total fat is in a serving of a food as well as what type of fat it is. Saturated and trans fats are the ones you want to limit, because we know they can be detrimental to digestive health, heart health, inflammation, and a host of other health issues. On the other hand, try to include monounsaturated and polyunsaturated fats, as they are both healthy fats that can help promote good gut health and overall health. Some labels will list the healthier fats separately; some will not. You can take a look at the total grams of fat and subtract the grams of saturated fat to get an idea of how much healthy fat is in there.

Get enough of certain nutrients

The nutrients listed next on the label are nutrients that most Americans *don't* get enough of and, therefore, need more in their daily diet. These nutrients include dietary fiber, vitamin A, vitamin C, calcium, and iron. The goal is to get at least 100% or more of your daily value for each (more on this later). Eating enough of these nutrients can help improve health and reduce the risk of some conditions and diseases. (Note that this is not a complete list, but the ones that the FDA feels are most needed.)

Watch total carbohydrates

Because all carbohydrates have some effect on digestive health, this is an important section on the food label. Total carbohydrates include complex carbs (starches), simple sugars, sugar alcohols, and dietary fiber. Although you can't isolate added sugar from naturally occurring sugars on a food label, it is still helpful to calculate the calories from total sugar. To do this, multiply grams of sugar by 4 (because there are 4 calories per 1 gram of sugar). For example, if a product contains 10 grams of sugar per serving, 40 calories of each serving come from sugar. If the product has no fruit or milk ingredients, it's a good bet that all of those calories are coming from added sugars. If you want more information on what kind(s) of sugar you're dealing with, you'll need to look at the ingredient list. You can also use label claims found on the front of the packaged food to help clue you in to how much sugar is in a product. Refer to Chapter 3 for more information on added sugars. Some examples of label claims:

- **"Sugar-free"**: less than 0.5 grams of sugar per serving.

- **"Reduced sugar"** or **"less sugar"**: at least 25 percent less sugar per serving compared to the same serving size of the original variety.

- **"No added sugar"** or **"without added sugar(s)"**: no sugar or sugar-containing ingredients such as juice or dried fruit are added during processing.

- Note that **"low sugar"** is not defined or allowed as a nutrient claim on a food label.

Your Nutrition Solution Tidbit: In 2014, the FDA proposed updates to the nutrition facts label on packaged foods. One of those proposed changes includes adding more information on added sugar so that consumers will be able to differentiate between added and natural sugar on the label. Stayed tuned for updates.

Figure out percent daily value

If you are not sure whether a food is high or low in the nutrients mentioned previously, the percent daily value (%DV) is a tool on the label that can help you figure that out. Start with the footnote on the bottom of the label, which tells you that all %DV's are based on a 2,000-calorie diet. This statement must appear on all food labels and does not change from product to product as the rest of the information may. This information is recommended dietary advice for all Americans and is not specific to the food product.

* Percent Daily Values are based on a 2,000 calorie diet. Your Daily Values may be higher or lower depending on your calorie needs.			
	Calories:	2,000	2,500
Total Fat	Less than	65g	80g
Sat Fat	Less than	20g	25g
Cholesterol	Less than	300mg	300mg
Sodium	Less than	2,400mg	2,400mg
Total Carbohydrate		300g	375g
Dietary Fiber		25g	30g

The recommendations for total fat, saturated fat, carbohydrates, and fiber are all based on a 2,000-calorie diet.

If you eat less than or more than the calorie levels used you need to adjust the recommended dietary advice to fit your individual needs. Cholesterol and sodium recommendations are the same no matter what calorie level you are consuming. The following is a chart of how the Percent Daily Values needs to be adjusted according to calorie level:

Adjusted Percent Daily Values for Specific Calorie Levels	
Calories	Adjusted %DV
1,200	60 percent
1,400	70 percent
1,600	80 percent
2,000	100 percent
2,200	110 percent
2,500	125 percent
2,800	140 percent
3,200	160 percent

Put %DV to use.

Now that you know what the daily values are, you can determine percent daily value (%DV), which will help you decide whether a food is high or low in a nutrient and, ultimately, if it is a smart food to choose. The %DV is listed to the right of most of the nutrients on the top part of the label. To help you decide quickly, use this guide:

- **5% DV or less** is considered low for that nutrient.
- **20% DV or more** is considered high for that nutrient.

You can use %DV not only to figure out if a food is high or low in a particular nutrient, but also to compare products. You can easily compare one product or brand to a similar product to make the better choice. When you compare, make sure that serving sizes are similar. Serving sizes are generally kept consistent for similar types of foods to make comparing them easier for the consumer.

You can also use %DV to help you make dietary trade-offs with other foods throughout the day. This allows you to eat even your favorite foods on occasion, and still fit them into a healthy gut diet. For instance, when one of your favorite foods is high in fat, you can balance it with foods that are lower in fat at other times of the day. But pay attention to how much of that favorite food you eat, so that the total amount of fat for your day stays below the 100%DV. If it is high in saturated or trans fat, eat it only on occasion.

One more way to use %DV is to help you distinguish one dietary claim from another, such as "light" versus "re-duced fat." Compare the %DV's for the nutrient in each of the foods to determine which one is higher or lower in that nutrient. This way there is no need to memorize all of the definitions that go along with those claims.

Read the additional nutrient information

The label also provides %DVs for a few essential vi-tamins and minerals, including, at minimum, vitamins A and C, calcium, and iron. Use the %DV so that you know how much one serving of a food contributes to the total amount you need per day.

Average* daily values used for these for nutrients are as follows:

- Vitamin A: 5,000 IU
- Vitamin C: 60 mg
- Calcium: 1,000 mg
- Iron: 18 mg

*For certain populations some of these numbers may be higher or lower.

For example, if calcium is listed as 25% DV, then one serving of that food will provide you with 25 percent of what you need for the day, or 250 mg.

Always check labels, and don't make assumptions. Just because yogurt is supposed to be a good calcium source doesn't mean you'll get the same amount in every yogurt. That goes for "live and active cultures" in yogurts, as well. Before you buy, compare brands and choose the ones that have the most calcium and protein, the lowest sugar and fat content, and that specifically state "contains live and active cultures" on the label. The point is to use the nutrition facts on food labels, as they are there to help you make better choices.

Your Nutrition Solution Tidbit: The %DVs for trans fat, sugar, and protein have yet not been established; however, you can still compare total amounts between brands to pick the better product.

Put It All Together

Once you have checked out all parts of the food label, you need to ask yourself whether the particular food is a smart choice. Does it fit into your healthy diet and weight-management plan? And, most importantly, does it fall into the healthy-gut category? Ask these questions to find out:

- Is one serving size enough for me, or do I need to double, triple, or even quadruple the carbs, calories, fat, and other nutrients on the label?

- Are the calories per serving low, moderate, or high? How many calories will be in the actual amount I eat?

- Are the nutrients that I need to limit, low, and are the nutrients I need more of, high?

- Is this food too high in fat, especially saturated or trans fat? Does this food contain any healthy fat?

- Does this food contain any added sugar, and if so, is it too much for my needs?

- Will this food provide me with enough fiber?

- Have I compared the label on this product to other brands of the same food to ensure I am getting the most nutritional bang for my buck? Should I look for an alternative?

Note that your answers to these questions may differ from those of another person, depending on calorie needs; whether you are trying to lose, maintain, or gain weight; nutritional goals; specific nutritional needs; and specific health issues, including digestive disorders. The bottom line is that the food label will enable you to compare foods based on key ingredients and therefore make better nutritional choices for a healthier and happier gut.

Nutrient Content Claims

Even if you don't have time to read each and every food label, something known as a "nutrient content claim" can help you find foods that meet your specific needs and goals quickly. According to the FDA, a nutrient content claim on a food package directly or by implication characterizes the level of a nutrient in a food. Examples include "low fat," "fat free," "high in fiber," and "reduced sugar." Each and every claim that is used on food packaging has a regulated definition. These are a few of the more popular ones that you may see on food packages:

- **"Reduced" or "less":** means at least 25 percent less calories, total fat, saturated fat, sugar, sodium, or cholesterol than the regular product. This doesn't necessarily mean the product is "low" in a nutrient if the regular product is quite high.

- **"Light" or "lite":** means the food contains one-third fewer calories or no more than half the fat of the regular or higher-calorie, higher-fat version; or no more than half the sodium of the higher-sodium version.

- **"Good source of," "contains," or "provides":** means the food contains between 10 to 19 percent of the daily value for a nutrient per serving.

- **"Excellent source of," "high in," or "rich in":** means the food contains 20 percent or more of the daily value for a nutrient per serving.

- **"More," "fortified," "enriched," "added," "extra," or "plus"**: means the food contains 10 percent or more of the daily value for a nutrient per serving, as compared to the regular product.
- **"Low fat"**: means 3 grams of fat or less per serving.
- **"Fat free"**: means less than 0.5 grams of fat per serving.
- **"Cholesterol free"**: means less than 2 milligrams cholesterol and 2 grams or less of saturated fat per serving.
- **"Low sodium"**: means 140 mg or less of sodium per serving.
- **"Sodium free"**: means less than 5 milligrams of sodium per serving.
- **"Low calorie"**: means 40 calories or less per serving.
- **"Calorie free"**: means less than 5 calories per serving.
- **"Lean" (on meat labels)**: means less than 10 grams of fat per serving, with 4.5 grams or less of saturated fat and 95 milligrams of cholesterol per serving.
- **"Extra lean" (on meat labels)**: means less than 5 grams of fat per serving, with less than 2 grams of saturated fat and 95 milligrams of cholesterol.

Health Claims

Health claims on labels are another tool to help you make healthier choices that are individualized to you and your specific health issues. According to the FDA, a health claim is any claim made on the label or in the labeling of a food, including dietary supplements, that expressly or by implication (including "third party" references, written statements, symbols, or vignettes) characterizes the relationship of any substance to a disease or health-related condition. Implied health claims include those statements, symbols, vignettes, or other forms of communication that suggest, within the context in which they are presented, that a relationship exists between the presence or level of a substance in the food and a disease or health-related condition. Here are a few examples of health claims:

- "Diets rich in whole-grain foods and other plant foods and low in total fat, saturated fat, and cholesterol may help reduce the risk of heart disease."

- "Low-fat diets rich in fiber-containing grain products, fruits, and vegetables may reduce the risk of some types of cancer, a disease associated with many factors."

- "Low-fat diets rich in fiber-containing grain products, fruits, and vegetables may reduce the risk of some types of cancer, a disease associated with many factors."

- *To find all of the nutrient content claims and health claims, visit the FDA at *www.fda.gov.*

Allergen Listings

Because some digestive symptoms are caused by high allergen foods, it is important to understand that you can use food labels to detect whether a food contains a specific ingredient(s) that you might be allergic to, intolerant of, or sensitive to. In the United States, the FDA, under the Food Allergen Labeling and Consumer Protection Act (FALCPA), requires manufacturers to list the eight major food allergens. This act or law was enacted in 2004 and addresses labeling of all packaged foods regulated by the FDA. A *major food allergen* is an ingredient that falls in one of the following eight foods or food groups *or* an ingredient that contains protein derived from one of them:

- Milk
- Eggs
- Fish
- Crustacean shellfish
- Tree nuts
- Wheat
- Peanuts
- Soybeans

These eight major food allergens account for 90 percent of all food allergies. Labels have to list the type of allergen—for example, tree nut (almond)—or the type of crustacean shellfish—for example, crab or shrimp. Also listed are any ingredients that contain a protein from the eight major food allergens as well as any allergens found in flavorings, colorings, and/or other additives. FALCPA requires food allergens to be specified on the label no matter what the quantity, but only when they are contained as an ingredient.

Your Nutrition Solution Tidbit: Manufactures are not required to include warnings concerning food allergens and cross-contamination of food allergens accidently being introduced during manufacturing or packaging. This can spell trouble if you are very sensitive to a food allergen. However, many manufacturers tend to include warnings voluntarily, though not always in a clear manner. The FDA is working to make this kind of labeling more consistent so that it is easier for consumers to identify allergens with no worries. If you are in doubt and you have an allergy or sensitivity, call the manufacturer and/or check with your doctor.

Although gluten is not on the list of major allergens, many people are sensitive to gluten or have celiac disease, a chronic digestive disorder, and cannot consume any amount of gluten. Gluten is a protein found in wheat, barley, and rye and is found in many foods and food ingredients. The good news is that the FDA has established a ruling defining guidelines for the use of the term "gluten free" on packaged food labels. This will greatly help those who need to live gluten-free be confident that items labeled "gluten-free" truly meet a defined standard for gluten content. The new ruling states that any food labeled "gluten free" must contain less than 20 parts per million of that protein.

The bottom line is if you have food allergies, intolerances, or sensitivities that you know are digestive triggers for you, be aware of what you are eating and drinking and be sure to check food labels and packaging. Even if that food was safe to eat the last time you bought it, check again, because manufacturers change their ingredients often. If you have any doubt, contact the manufacturer about whether the food contains a specific allergen, including gluten.

chapter 6

14-day menu guide and stocking your kitchen

So far you've been provided with a great deal of information that will help you start using nutrition as a large part of both promoting a healthier gut and managing existing digestive disorders. This chapter will help you to put it all together by providing 14 days of easy-to-follow menus to get you started on the right foot. You can use these menus as a starting point to help you plan your own menus according to your individual likes and dislikes. In addition, this chapter will provide you with an extensive list of foods and beverages that are great to have on hand in order to keep your gut healthy and happy.

14-Day Menu Guide

The following menus are chock full of gut healthy foods and void of the foods that are commonly considered gut-busters. Portion sizes will need to be adjusted depending on your individual caloric need and your weight loss/maintenance goals. The menus are low in saturated fat, trans fat, cholesterol, and refined sugar, and moderate in sodium. They are rich in healthy fats and provide plenty of fiber and nutrients essential for proper digestive functioning. Make sure you substitute any foods that are personal triggers. The format of these menus follows the recommendation of frequent and smaller meals for plenty of opportunities to get your food groups in, keep your hunger satisfied, and keep your metabolism chugging along throughout day. If you get hungry after dinner, snack on fruit, yogurt, nuts, seeds, light popcorn, whole-grain crackers, and so on. Don't forget to drink plenty of water throughout your day, as well.

Your Nutrition Solution Tidbit: Sufficient water intake throughout the day is vital. Staying hydrated is essential for good health and just about every function in your body, especially your digestion. Water is important for regular bowel movements, which is important for good colon health.

Day 1

Breakfast

Steel-cut oatmeal, cooked with water

Top with raspberries, chopped walnuts, dash cinnamon, and light almond milk

Kombucha tea

AM Snack

Apple slices dipped in almond butter

Cranberry juice (100% juice)

Lunch

Wrap:

Chicken breast, skinless, cooked, diced

Mashed avocado

Baby spinach leaves and diced tomato

Whole-wheat tortilla or whole-wheat pita

Seedless, red or green grapes, or sliced strawberries on the side

PM Snack

Kefir

Rice cakes, brown rice

Dinner

Salmon, wild-caught, grilled or baked (marinate with light teriyaki sauce, extra-virgin olive oil, and a few shakes of ground ginger for a few hours before cooking)

Steamed fresh asparagus, drizzled with extra-virgin olive oil

Brown rice mixed with salsa, beans, and a few shakes of cumin

Day 2

Breakfast

Whole-grain English muffin, toasted

Almond butter

Cantaloupe, cubed

Turkey sausage links, cooked

Soymilk, light

AM Snack

Greek yogurt, non-fat, with "live and active cultures," mixed with 1 Tbsp. ground flaxseed and blueberries

Lunch

Sandwich:

Fresh turkey breast or nitrate-free deli meat with

Mashed avocado or guacamole, spinach leaves, sliced tomato, in whole-wheat pita

Baby carrots

Celery stalks, trimmed

Kombucha tea

PM Snack

Grapes, seedless, red or green

Almond milk, light

Dinner

Skinless, chicken breast, baked, broiled or grilled

Broccoli, steamed

Jerusalem artichoke, baked, with 1 Tbsp. non–trans fat margarine

Dark leafy green salad topped with extra-virgin olive oil, balsamic vinegar, and a dash of lemon

Green tea

Day 3

Breakfast

Bran cereal (check sugar content) topped with

Blueberries and fat-free milk

Banana

Kombucha tea

AM Snack

Cottage cheese, low-fat, topped with

Ground cinnamon and sliced peaches

Cranberry juice (100% juice)

Lunch

Salad:

Romaine lettuce with fresh vegetables such as red peppers, broccoli, and cucumbers, topped with garbanzo beans, sunflower seeds, chopped cooked egg whites, tossed with extra-virgin olive oil, balsamic vinegar, and a pinch of cumin as dressing

PM Snack

Hummus and baby carrots/celery sticks

Kefir

Dinner

Stir-fry:

Shrimp, shelled, deveined

Edamame

Red pepper

Onion

Water chestnuts

Ground or grated ginger

Soy sauce

Minced garlic

Extra-virgin olive oil

Cooked brown rice or whole-grain couscous

Day 4

Breakfast

Steel-cut oatmeal, cooked with water, topped with

Ground cinnamon and raisins

1 pear

Soymilk, light

Green tea

AM Snack

Smoothie:

1 banana

Cranberries

Soymilk (light)

1 Tbsp. ground flaxseed

Use frozen fruit or add protein powder to make the smoothie thicker

Lunch

Tuna salad wrap:

3 oz. tuna, canned in water, mixed with

1 1/2 Tbsp. Greek yogurt, non-fat (with "live and active cultures), 1 1/2 Tbsp. mashed avocado, 1 Tbsp. diced celery, 1 tsp. Dijon mustard, and garlic powder to taste

Roll tuna salad in whole-wheat tortilla

Vegetable soup, low-sodium

1 apple

PM Snack

Guacamole (for a twist try adding quinoa, a whole grain)

Fresh vegetables for dipping

Kombucha tea

Dinner

Mix together:

1 1/2 cups pasta, whole wheat, cooked

1/2 cup black beans, canned, drained

1/2 cup carrots, steamed

1/4 cup peas, steamed

1/2 cup zucchini, streamed

1/2 Tbsp. extra-virgin olive oil plus 2 Tbsp. freshly grated Parmesan cheese

Dark leafy green salad with raw vegetables, tossed with extra-virgin olive oil, balsamic vinegar, and a bit of lemon juice

Day 5

Breakfast

Bagel, whole grain

Almond butter

Strawberries or blueberries

Kombucha tea

AM Snack

Smoothie:

Cranberries

Soymilk, light

1 Tbsp. ground flaxseed

Use frozen fruit or protein powder to make the smoothie thicker

Lunch

Veggie wrap:

Diced tomato

Baby spinach

Canned black beans

Diced avocado

Whole-wheat tortilla

Celery and carrot sticks

Orange

PM Snack

Handful of almonds and raisins

Kefir

Dinner

Skinless chicken breast marinated in lemon and coriander, grilled or baked

Wild rice, cooked

Asparagus, steamed

Day 6

Breakfast

Whole-grain waffle

Peanut butter

Cantaloupe, cubed

Orange juice, 100% juice, calcium fortified

AM Snack

Handful of walnuts

Grapefruit

Green tea

Lunch

Soup:

Lentil, low-sodium (sprinkle cayenne pepper for a kick)

6 whole-wheat crackers

1 Pear

PM Snack

Popcorn, plain or light

Dinner

Halibut, wild caught; broiled, baked, or grilled (marinate it ahead of time with soy sauce, extra-virgin olive oil, and sprinkle with ginger and garlic)

Whole-grain couscous, cooked and mixed with salsa and black beans

Spinach, steamed

Day 7

Breakfast

Egg whites scrambled with fresh sliced mushrooms, diced tomatoes, and chopped spinach

Whole-wheat toast topped with almond butter

Strawberries, sliced

Cranberry juice (100% juice)

AM Snack

Apple spread with peanut butter

Lunch

Wrap: Skinless chicken breast, cooked, diced

Garbanzo beans

Diced tomato

Sliced avocado

Salsa

Whole-wheat tortilla

Cottage cheese, low-fat, sprinkled with ground cinnamon and topped with slieced peaches

PM Snack

Hummus

Fresh raw vegetables for dipping

Kombucha tea

Dinner

Burger:

Extra-lean ground turkey

Whole-grain pita

Sliced avocado

Sliced tomato

Spinach leaves

Sauerkraut, rinsed and warmed (refrigerated, not canned)

Dark leafy green salad with raw vegetables, tossed with extra-virgin olive oil, balsamic vinegar, and lemon

Day 8

Breakfast

Steel-cut oatmeal, cooked

Chopped walnuts

Blueberries

Soymilk, light

Ground cinnamon

Grapefruit

AM Snack

Smoothie, mix in a blender:

1/2 banana

1/2 cup blackberries, frozen, no sugar added

1/2 cup Greek yogurt, non-fat, plain (with "live and active cultures")

1 cup soymilk, light

1 Tbsp. honey

1/4 cup ice

Lunch

Black bean soup, low-sodium

Whole-grain crackers

Cantaloupe, diced

Kombucha tea

PM Snack

Handful of almonds and raisins

Kefir

Dinner

Salmon (wild caught), baked, sprinkled with garlic

Roasted butternut squash drizzled with cinnamon and extra-virgin olive oil

Broccoli, steamed

Day 9

Breakfast

Whole-grain English muffin

Almond butter

Canadian bacon or turkey bacon, cooked

Hard-boiled egg

Cantaloupe, diced

AM Snack

Greek yogurt, non-fat (with "live and active cultures")

1 Tbsp. ground flaxseed and pinch of ground cinnamon

Lunch

3 oz. tuna, canned in water, mixed with

1 1/2 Tbsp. Greek yogurt, non-fat

1 1/2 Tbsp. mashed avocado

1 Tbsp. diced celery

1 tsp. Dijon mustard

Garlic powder to taste

Whole-grain crackers

Lentil soup, low-sodium

PM Snack

Popcorn, plain or light

1 apple

Green tea

Dinner

Skinless, chicken breast, grilled

Sautéed mushrooms and zucchini, tossed in extra-virgin olive oil and minced garlic, mixed into

Whole-grain spaghetti, cooked

Fresh parmesan cheese

Romaine salad with fresh vegetables, topped with extra-virgin olive oil, vinegar, lemon, pinch of cumin

Day 10

Breakfast

Bran cereal (check for sugar content)

Fat-free milk

Sliced strawberries

Orange juice, 100% juice, calcium fortified

AM Snack

Handful of raisins and walnuts

Cranberry juice (100% juice)

Kefir

Lunch

Hard-boiled egg

Cottage cheese with blueberries and ground cinnamon

Kombucha tea

PM Snack

Smoothie, mix in blender:

1/2 cup blackberries, frozen

1/2 cup Greek yogurt, non-fat, plain (with "live and active cultures")

1 cups soymilk, light

1 Tbsp. honey

1/4 tsp. ginger root, finely grated

Dinner

Trout, baked

Cauliflower, steamed and sprinkled with cumin

Spinach, steamed

Jerusalem artichoke, baked with non–trans fat margarine

Day 11

Breakfast

Cooked quinoa, topped with ground cinnamon, blue-berries, and walnuts

Soymilk, light

Kombucha tea

AM Snack

Smoothie made with:

Banana

Cranberries, unsweetened

Almond milk, light

1 Tbsp. ground flaxseed

Use frozen fruit and/or protein powder to make the smoothie thicker

Lunch

Romaine lettuce salad with fresh vegetables such as broccoli, red onions, and cucumbers

Top with garbanzo beans, pumpkin seeds, chopped cooked egg whites

Toss with extra-virgin olive oil, balsamic vinegar, lemon juice

Whole-wheat crackers

Green tea

PM Snack

Hummus

Raw cauliflower

Kefir

Dinner

Turkey kielbasa, baked, broiled, or grilled

Sauerkraut, rinsed and warmed (refrigerated, not canned)

Sweet potato French fries, oven baked

1 cup broccoli, steamed

Day 12

Breakfast

Breakfast sandwich:

Egg whites scrambled

Goat cheese

Canadian bacon, cooked

English muffin, whole-grain, toasted

Grapefruit

AM Snack

1 apple

Almond butter

Cranberry juice (100% juice)

Lunch

Vegetable and barley soup, low-sodium (add some cayenne pepper for a kick)

Dark leafy green salad with fresh vegetables, topped with extra-virgin olive oil, vinegar, and lemon

PM Snack

Trail mix made from almonds, dried cranberries, raisins

Kefir

Dinner

Turkey meatballs, made with extra-lean turkey breast

Spaghetti, whole-grain

Spaghetti sauce, homemade

Dark leafy green salad with fresh vegetables, topped with extra-virgin olive oil, vinegar, and lemon

Day 13

Breakfast

Cooked quinoa, topped with ground cinnamon and blackberries

Almond milk, light

Kombucha tea

AM Snack

Rice cakes, brown

Almond butter

Grapes, seedless, red or white

Lunch

Barley salad:

Cooked barley

Your favorite cooked vegetables

Beans

Tofu

Green tea

PM Snack

Tart cherries

Walnuts

Dinner

Pork tenderloin, baked or grilled

Oven-steamed spaghetti squash, drizzled with extra-virgin olive oil

Zucchini, steamed

Day 14

Breakfast

Whole-grain English muffin

Almond butter and honey

Grapefruit

Kombucha tea

AM Snack

Greek or soy yogurt, non-fat ("with live and active cultures")

1 Tbsp. flaxseed

Mixed berries

Eat as-is or use frozen mixed berries and blend for a smoothie

Lunch

Chili:

Extra-lean ground turkey

Kidney beans

Onion

Tomato sauce

Pinch of turmeric, garlic, cumin, and other spices. Add cayenne pepper if you want to heat it up.

Dark leafy green salad with fresh vegetables, topped with extra-virgin olive oil, vinegar, and lemon

PM Snack

Brown rice cakes

Almond butter

Walnuts

Dried cranberries

Dinner

Salmon, grilled or baked, topped with mango salsa

Fresh asparagus, steamed

Cauliflower, steamed

Your Nutrition Solution Tidbit: Kombucha tea is a lightly effervescent drink made by adding good bacteria and yeast to sugar and black or green tea and allowing it to ferment. The resulting fermented tea is beneficial to the gut.

Stocking Your Kitchen

A well-stocked kitchen with plenty of gut-friendly foods will make life much easier. When you know you can grab a snack or a quick meal with the foods you have on hand, you will relieve some of your stress and anxiety about keeping your gut healthier and managing any GI symptoms. You might just find that your whole family will eat healthier once you have your kitchen stocked properly! This is just a sampling of foods to get you started; there are many more you can add. Keep in mind that you may need to adjust this list for any foods that you are allergic to, intolerant of, or sensitive to, or any foods that cause you trouble. This is far from an exhaustive list of foods that are gut healthy, but it will give you a good jumping-off point.

Fruit (Fresh, frozen, or canned in its own juice/ organic when possible)

- Apples
- Apricots
- Avocados
- Bananas
- Blackberries
- Blueberries
- Cantaloupe
- Cherries (especially tart cherries)
- Cranberries
- Grapefruit
- Grapes
- Kiwi
- Lemons
- Limes
- Mangoes
- Oranges
- Peaches
- Pear
- Pineapple
- Plums
- Prunes

- Raisins
- Raspberries
- Strawberries
- Watermelon

Vegetables (Fresh, frozen, or canned with low or no salt/organic when possible)

- Asparagus
- Beets
- Bell peppers (green, red, orange, and yellow)
- Broccoli
- Brussel's sprouts
- Cabbage (red or green)
- Carrots
- Cauliflower
- Celery
- Corn
- Green Beans
- Jerusalem artichoke
- Kale
- Mushrooms
- Onions
- Peas
- Potatoes
- Radishes
- Romaine lettuce

- Sauerkraut
- Scallions
- Spinach
- Squash (summer or winter)
- Sweet potatoes
- Swiss chard
- Tomatoes
- Zucchini

Grains

- Amaranth
- Barley
- Brown rice
- Buckwheat
- Bulgur
- Couscous, whole grain
- Kamut
- Millet
- Oatmeal (old fashioned or steel cut)
- Popcorn (light)
- Quinoa
- Whole-grain/whole-wheat breads, pitas, tortillas, rolls
- Whole-wheat pasta
- Whole-grain crackers
- Wild rice

Fish/shellfish (freeze until needed)

- Cod
- Flounder
- Halibut
- Mackerel
- Mussels
- Oysters
- Salmon (wild)
- Sardines (canned in olive oil or water)
- Shrimp
- Trout
- Tuna (canned in water)

Protein and Meat (grass fed when possible/freeze until needed)

- Beef, lean, grass fed
- Chicken breast, skinless
- Eggs/egg whites
- Pork tenderloin
- Tempeh
- Tofu
- Turkey breast, skinless
- Turkey breast, ground

Dairy Products

- Almond milk, light
- Fat-free milk

- Greek yogurt, non-fat, light (with "live and active cultures")
- Kefir
- Rice milk
- Soymilk, light

Herbs and spices (fresh or dried)

- Allspice
- Basil
- Bay leaf
- Cayenne pepper
- Cilantro
- Cinnamon
- Coriander
- Curry powder
- Cumin
- Clove
- Dill
- Fennel
- Garlic (powder and minced)
- Ginger
- Mustard
- Nutmeg
- Paprika
- Parsley
- Pepper (black and/or red)

- Peppermint
- Rosemary
- Saffron
- Sage
- Tarragon
- Thyme
- Turmeric

Legumes, Nuts, and Seeds

- Almonds
- Black beans
- Cashews
- Chia seeds
- Flaxseed (whole or ground)
- Garbanzo beans (chickpeas)
- Kidney beans
- Lentils
- Navy beans
- Peanuts
- Pine nuts
- Pinto beans
- Pumpkin seeds
- Sesame seeds
- Soybeans/edamame
- Split peas
- Sunflower seeds
- Walnuts

Oils/Fats

- Canola oil
- Evening primrose oil
- Extra-virgin olive oil
- Grapeseed oil
- Nut butters (such as almond butter)
- Peanut butter
- Walnut oil

Miscellaneous Items

- Apple cider vinegar
- Chocolate, dark, plain
- Green tea
- Guacamole
- Honey
- Hummus
- Kombucha tea
- Miso
- Red wine
- Soy sauce

your best resources

Websites

National Institutes of Health/Human Microbiome Project: *http://commonfund.nih.gov/hmp/index*

Healthline/Peptic Ulcers: *www.healthline.com/health/peptic-ulcer#Overview1*

WebMD/Digestive Disorders Health Center: *www.webmd.com/digestive-disorders/default.htm*

WebMD/Digestive Health Center: *www.webmd.boots.com/digestive-disorders/small-intestinal-bacteria-sibo*

American Gastroenterological Association: *www.gastro.org/*

Celiac Disease Foundation: *http://celiac.org/*

The University of Chicago/Celiac Disease Center: *www.cureceliacdisease.org/*

National Institute of Diabetes and Digestive and Kidney Diseases: *www.niddk.nih.gov/Pages/default.aspx*

Nutrition.gov (Herbal Supplements): *www.nutrition.gov/dietary-supplements/herbal-supplements*

University of Maryland Medical Center: *http://umm.edu/*

American Heart Association: *www.heart.org*

Academy of Nutrition and Dietetics: *www.eatright.org*

USDA Choosemyplate.gov: *www.choosemyplate.gov*

Clean Eating: *www.cleaneatingmag.com/*

Environmental Working Group: *www.ewg.org/*

U.S. FDA Good Allergies: *www.fda.gov/Food/Resources ForYou/Consumers/ucm079311.htm*

U.S. Food and Drug Administration: *www.fda.gov*

Dietary Guidelines for Americans, 2010: *www.health.gov/ dietaryguidelines*

U.S. Department of Health and Human Services. Physical Activity Guidelines for Americans: *www.health.gov/paguidelines/*

Whole Grains Council: *http://wholegrainscouncil.org*

The World's Healthiest Foods: *www.whfoods.com/*

Certified LEAP Therapists/Dietitians*

Oxford Biomedical Technologies: *http://nowleap.com/*

Find a Certified LEAP Therapist: 888-Now-LEAP (toll free) or 561-848-7111

*Many of these dietitians will counsel patients by phone.

Jan Patenaude, RD, CLT

Director of Medical Nutrition, Oxford Biomedical Technologies, Inc., Riviera Beach, Florida

888-now-leap.com OR Toll free 888-669-5327

Telecommuting Nationwide

Jan@CertifiedLEAPTherapist.com

http://CertifiedLEAPTherapist.com

http://PINTEREST.com/LEAPMRT

www.facebook.com/LEAP.MRT

Twitter: @LEAPMRT

Michal Hogan, RD, LD, CLT

LEAP Mentor, Author of *Food Sensitivity* series, *Tactical Reimbursement*

Nutrition Results, LLC

Easton Executive Suites

4200 Regent Street, Suite 200

Columbus, Ohio 43219

www.meg-enterprises.com/classes/food-sensitivity-series

Phone: (614) 944-5123 Fax (614) 987-8520

Dianne Rishikof, MS, RDN, LDN

Nutrition Consulting, Gut Health

www.diannerishikof.com

dianne.rishikof@gmail.com

www.facebook.com/diannerishikof.nutrition

https://twitter.com/DianneRishikof

www.pinterest.com/diannerish/

Alexandra Caspero, RD

Certified LEAP Therapist

Delish Knowledge

www.delishknowledge.com

alexandra.caspero@gmail.com

Patsy Catsos, MS, RDN, LD

Author of *IBS—Free at Last!* and the *Flavor Without FODMAPs* cookbooks

Editor of IBSFree.net

www.facebook.com/ibsfree

www.Pinterest.com/pcatsos

Twitter: @CatsosIBSFreeRD

Sarah R. Lippman, MS RD

Registered Dietitian Nutritionist

http://www.thefunctionalnutritionist.com

sarah@thefunctionalnutritionist.com

Niki Strealy, RDN, LD

Nutrition Entrepreneurs Director-Elect Member Services

www.DiarrheaDietitian.com

Strategic Nutrition, LLC

Twitter: @DiarrheaRD

(503) 974-6454

Bonnie R. Giller, MS, RD, CDN, CDE

Medical Nutrition Therapist, Certified Intuitive Eating Counselor

BRG Dietetics & Nutrition, P.C.

516-486-4569

bonnie@BRGhealth.com

http://www.BRGhealth.com

http://www.DietFreeZone.com: Get Your Free e-Book "5 Steps to a Body You Love Without Dieting"

Facebook.com/BRGDieteticsandNutritionPC

Twitter.com/brghealth

Pinterest.com/bgiller

Websites:

Brghealth.com: Eat Intelligently. Be Mindful. Nourish Your Body.

DietFreeZone.com: Enjoy the Freedom to Eat While Getting the Body You Love.

PassoverTheHealthyWay.com: Passover *Can* be Easy and Healthy.

www.DietFreeZone.com: Get Your Free Guide "5 Steps to a Body You Love without Dieting"

Blogs:

The Nutrition Key with BRG: *http://brghealth.com/ category/the-nutrition-key-with-brg-blog/*

iEat Mindfully Intuitive Eating: *http://brghealth.com/ category/ieat-mindfully/*

Social Media:

www.facebook.com/BRGDieteticsandNutritionPC

https://twitter.com/brghealth

www.linkedin.com/in/bonniegiller

www.pinterest.com/bgiller/

Gita Patel MS RDN CDE CLT LD

Feedinghealth

gita@feedinghealth.com

www.feedinghealth.com

Nancy Mazarin MS, RDN, CDN

891 Northern Boulevard, Suite 204

Great Neck, N.Y. 11021

(516) 466-9087

nmeatrite@mazarinrd.com

http://mazarinrd.com

Sandy Livingston, RD, LD/N

800 Village Square Crossing, Suite 209

Palm Beach Gardens, Fl. 33410

sandy@palmbeachnutritionist.com

www.palmbeachnutritionist.com

(561) 371-5105

Kate Scarlata, RDN

Digestive health and FODMAP expert

www.katescarlata.com

Lori Sullivan Nutrition

Offices in South Windsor and West Hartford, Connecticut

Lori@LoriSullivanNutrition.com

www.LoriSullivanNutrition.com

(800) 658-0512

Most insurances accepted.

bibliography

(For additional sources, please visit *www.nutrifocus.net*.)

Abou-Donia M.B., El-Masry E.M., Abdel-Rahman A.A., McLendon R.E., and Schiffman S.S. "Splenda Alters Gut Microflora and Increases Intestinal P-glycoprotein and Cytochrome P-450 in Male Rats." *Journal of Toxicology and Environmental Health* 71.21 (2008): 1415–429. *National Center for Biotechnology Information*. U.S. National Library of Medicine/PubMed.gov.

Baumler, Megan D. "Gut Bacteria." *Today's Dietitian* 15.6 (2013): 46. *Gut Bacteria*. November 2014.

Bode, C., and C.J. Bode, MD. "Alcohol's Role in Gastrointestinal Tract Disorders." *Alcohol Health and Research World* 1.1 (1997): 76–83.

Cho, Ilseung, and Martin J. Blaser. "The Human Microbiome: At the Interface of Health and Disease." *The Human Microbiome: At the Interface of Health and Disease* 13.4 (2012): 260–70. *Nature Reviews. Genetics*. U.S. National Library of Medicine. March 13, 2012.

"Cranberries." The World's Healthiest Foods. N.p., n.d.

"Cranberry." National Center for Complementary and Integrative Health. U.S. Dept. of Health and Human Services, April 2012.

Dahm, Robin B. "Resistant Carbohydrates in Dry Beans: Friend of Colonic Probiotics, Foe of Colorectal Cancer. See more at: *http://beaninstitute.com/*

resistant-carbohydrates-in-dry-beans-friend-of-colonic-probiotics-foe-of-colorectal-cancer/#sthash.BHMRPtRZ.dpuf." *The Bean Institute.* N.p., n.d.

DiBaise, John K., and Amy Foxx-Orenstein. "Obesity." *American College of Gastroenterology.* N.p., April 2010.

"Digestive Diseases Statistics for the United States." Digestive Diseases Statistics for the United States. N.p., September 2013.

Elinav, Eran. "Gut Bacteria, Artificial Sweeteners, and Glucose Intolerance." *American Committee for the Weizmann Institute of Science.* N.p., 17 September 2014.

"Exercise May Spur More Varied Gut Microbes, Study Finds." WebMD News from HealthDay. WebMD, 2013.

Duncan, Sylvia H., Alvaro Belenguer, Grietje Holtrop, Alexandra M. Johnstone, Harry J. Flint, and Gerald E. Lobley. "Reduced Dietary Intake of Carbohydrates by Obese Subjects Results in Decreased Concentrations of Butyrate and Butyrate-Producing Bacteria in Feces." *Applied and Environmental Microbiology* 73.4 (2007): 1073–078.

"Guidance for Industry: A Food Labeling Guide (6. Ingredient Lists)." U.S. Food and Drug Administration. N.p., February 2013.

"Intestinal Gas from Complex Carbohydrates or Lactose Intolerance." Gastrointestinal Society. Canadian Society of Intestinal Research, February 2001.

Kaur, N., and A.K. Gupta. "Applications of Inulin and Oligofructose in Health and Nutrition." *Journal of Biosciences* 27.7 (202): 703–14. *National Center for Biotechnology Information.* U.S. National Library of Medicine/PubMed.gov.

Keller, Maur. "A Bounty of Alternative Whole Grains." *Today's Dietitian* 13.11 (2011): 28. *Today's Dietitian.*

———. "Healthier Frozen Foods." *Today's Dietitian* 14.10 (2012): 36. *Today's Dietitian.*

Lesbros-Pantoflickova, Drahoslava, Irène Corthésy-Theulaz, and André L. Blum. "Helicobacter Pylori and Probiotics." *The Journal of Nutrition* 137.3 (2007): 8125–185. American Society for Nutrition.

Leung, Lawrence, Taylor Riutta, Jyoti Kotecha, and Walter Rosser. "Chronic Constipation: An Evidence-Based Review." *Journal of the American Board of Family Medicine* 24.4 (2011): 436–51. Jabfm.org. Accessed December 10, 2014.

Mahmood, A., A. J. FitzGerald, T. Marchbank, E. Ntatsaki, D. Murray, S. Ghosh, and R. J. Playford. "Zinc Carnosine, a Health Food Supplement That Stabilizes Small Bowel Integrity and Stimulates Gut Repair Processes." *Gut* 56.2 (2007): 168–75.

"Proposed Changes to the Nutrition Facts Label." U.S. Food and Drug Administration. N.p., 1 August 2014.

Richards, Byron J. "How Imbalanced Digestive Bacteria Cause Obesity and Heart Disease." *Wellness Resources.* 20 May 2013.

Robert A. Koeth, Zeneng Wang, Bruce S. Levison, Jennifer A. Buffa,, Elin Org, Brendan T. Sheehy, Earl B. Britt, Xiaoming Fu, Yuping Wu, Lin Li, Jonathan D. Smith, Joseph A. DiDonato, Jun Chen, Hongzhe Li, Gary D. Wu, James D. Lewis, Manya Warrier, J. Mark Brown, Ronald M. Krauss, W.H. Wilson Tang, Frederic D. Bushman, Aldons J. Lusis, and Stanley L. Hazen. "Intestinal Microbiota Metabolism of L-carnitine, a

Nutrient in Red Meat, Promotes Atherosclerosis." *Nature Medicine* 19 (2013): 576–85. 7 Aprril 2013.

Satyanarayana, M.N. "Capsaicin and Gastric Ulcers." *Critical Reviews in Food Science and Nutrition* 46.4 (2006): 275–328. *National Center for Biotechnology Information.* U.S. National Library of Medicine/PubMed.gov.

Satyanarayana MN. "Capsaicin and Gastric Ulcers." *Critical Reviews in Food Science and Nutrition* 46.4 (2006): 275–328. *National Center for Biotechnology Information.* U.S. National Library of Medicine/ PubMed.gov. Accessed 28 January 2015.

Smith, Jeffery M. "Are Genetically Modified Foods a Gut-Wrenching Combination?" *Are Genetically Modified Foods a Gut-Wrenching Combination?* Institute for Responsible Technology, n.d.

Strate, L. L., Y. L. Liu, S. Syngal, W. H. Aldoori, and E. L. Giovannucci. "Nut, Corn, and Popcorn Consumption and the Incidence of Diverticular Disease." *JAMA: The Journal of the American Medical Association* 300.8 (2008): 907–14.

Van Der Hulst RR, Von Meyenfeldt MF, and Soeters PB. "Glutamine: An Essential Amino Acid for the Gut." *Nutrition* 12.11-12 (1996): 78–81. *National Center for Biotechnology Information.* U.S. National Library of Medicine/PubMed.gov.

Welsh, JA, A. Sharma, JL Abramson, V. Vaccarino, C. Gillespie, and MB Vos. "Caloric Sweetener Consumption and Dyslipidemia among US Adults." *Journal of the American Medical Association* 303.15 (2010): 1490–497. *National Center for Biotechnology Information.* U.S. National Library of Medicine/PubMed.gov.

index

abdominal
bloating, SIBO and, 43
pain, SIBO and, 43
acacia fiber, 91
acid
production, excessive, 24
reflux, 39
active, the importance of staying physically, 113-114
added sugar, identifying, 92-97
additional nutrient information, reading the, 172-173
alcohol,
excessive intake of, 24
sugar, 129
the benefits of avoiding, 124-125
allergen listings, 177-180
allergies, food, 65-66
artificial sweeteners, 128-129
asparagus, the benefits of, 139-140
bacteria,
disease and, 21-22
gut, 19-21
H.pylori, 24-25
sugar and, 93
bananas, the benefits of, 139-140
black beans, the benefits of, 141-143

blueberries, the benefits of, 143-144
BMI, calculating your, 106-107
calories, focusing on, 167
carbohydrates,
the relationship with, 48
watching total, 169-170
cayenne pepper, the benefits of, 146
celiac disease, 72-75
cereals, sugary, 132-133
cleaner eating, committing to, 80-86
coffee, the benefits of avoiding, 124-125
colitis, 39
constipation,
chronic, 29-32
SIBO and, 44
coriander, the benefits of, 144-145
cranberries, the benefits of, 137-138
cravings for sugar, how to control, 94-95
Crohn's disease, 39
probiotics and, 60
cumin, the benefits of, 145-146
deficiencies, vitamin, 44

detox diet, helping your gut with a, 45-46

diarrhea, SIBO and, 43

dietary gut supplements, 58-65

digestive enzymes, 62-63

disaccharides, 77

discretionary calories, 93-94

disease, gut bacteria and, 21-22

diseases, the gut and associated, 23-39

diverticular disease, 27-29

duodenal ulcers, 23

emotional symptoms, gut health and, 22

enzymes, digestive, 62-63

esophageal ulcers, 23

exercise, the importance of, 114-118

fad diets, the cons of, 109

family history, the significance of, 25

family, the importance of a supportive, 148

fast food, the benefits of avoiding, 126-127

fat, avoiding certain types of, 82-83

fats, consuming healthy, 83

fennel, the benefits of, 145

fiber
  intake, boosting your daily, 86-90
  supplements, 90-92

fiber,
  acacia, 91
  facts about, 53-56
  the importance of, 49-50

flatulence,
  excessive, 56-58
  SIBO and, 43

flaxseed, ground, the benefits of, 136-127

FODMAP diet, 69, 76-78

food
  allergies, 65-66
  intolerances, 66-69
  labels, the importance of, 164-175
  sensitivities, 69-70

foods to avoid, 122-133

foods to include in your diet, 133-146

frozen dinners, the benefits to avoiding, 130-132

fructose intolerance, 68-69

fruits, incorporating, 81-82

gallstones, 35-39

gas, SIBO and, 43

ginger, the benefits of, 144

glutamine, 63-64

gluten-free diet, 72-75

GMOs, the effects of, 41

goals, setting short- and long-term, 111

grains,
  reducing your intake of certain, 82
  understanding the difference between, 50-52

grass-fed beef, importance of choosing, 83

Greek yogurt, the benefits of, 134-135

H. pylori bacteria, 24-25

H. pylori, zinc carnosine and, 65

health
    claims, 176-177
    conditions, the gut and, 23-39
healthy fats, consuming, 83
healthy weight, reaching and maintaining a, 105-114
herbs and spices, gut-friendly, 144-146
high-fructose corn syrup, 123-124
IBS, 32-35
immunoglobulin, food allergies and, 65-66
inflammatory bowel disease, 38
ingredients, eating foods with only a few, 82
insoluble fiber, 55-56
intestinal flora, prebiotics and, 60
intolerance,
    fructose, 66-67
    lactose, 66-67
    overall food, 65-69
inulin, prebiotics and, 91
irritable bowel syndrome (see IBS)
Jerusalem artichoke, the benefits of, 140-141
kefir, the benefits of, 138-139
kidney disease, 25
kitchen, stocking your, 200-207
lactose intolerance, 66-67
leaky gut syndrome, 40-41
liver disease, 25
low carbohydrate diets, 50
low-density lipoproteins, prebiotics and, 60
mediator release test, 70-72
menu guide, 14-day, 182-200

menu planning tips, 148-154
microbiota, gut, 20-21
monosaccharides, 77
non-celiac gluten sensitivity, 75-76
nutrient content claims, 175-176
nutrients,
    getting enough of certain, 168
    limiting certain, 168
nutrition facts panel, 165
oatmeal, the benefits of, 136
obesity, 42
oligosaccharides, 77
ologofructose, prebiotics and, 91
organic foods, why you should eat, 83-85
overgrowth of bacteria in the gut, 44
painkillers, the gut and the usage of, 24
peptic ulcer disease, 23-27
percent daily value, figuring out, 170-172
polyols, 78
prebiotics, 60-61
    the importance of, 45
prescription medication, effects of, 24
probiotics, 59-60
    the importance of, 45
processed grains, reducing, 82
produce, the importance of, 155-157
psyllium, 91
radiation treatment, effects of, 25
recipes, incorporating new, 149-150

red meat, the benefits to avoiding, 130

refined
grains, 96
sugar, reducing, 82

saturated fat, avoiding, 82-83

sedentary lifestyle, 42

sensitivities, food, 69-70

SIBO, 42-43

small intestinal bacterial growth (see SIBO)

smoking, the effects of, 25

snacks, the importance of, 151-154

soft drinks, the benefits of avoiding, 127-128

soluble fiber, 54-55

starches, the gut and, 49

stomach cancer, 25

stress management, treating gut issues with, 45

stress,
chronic, 42
gut health and, 22
managing your, 118-120

sugar
alcohol, 129
cravings, how to control, 94-95

sugar,
different types of, 52-53
limiting added, 92-97
reducing your intake of, 82

sugars, overview of, 48-49

sugary cereals, avoiding, 132-133

supermarket, navigating the, 154-155

supplements, vitamin, 45

sweeteners, artificial, 128-129

tobacco, smoking and chewing, 25

trans fat, avoiding, 82-83

ulcers,
duodenal, 23
esophageal, 23

unhealthy gut,
causes of an, 42-45
symptoms of an, 22-23

vegetables, incorporating, 81-82

vitamin deficiencies, 44

water,
losing weight and drinking, 114
the essentials of drinking enough, 82

weight, reaching and maintaining a healthy, 105-114

white bread, avoiding, 122-123

whole grains, opting for, 97-104

yogurt, Greek, 134-135

zinc carnosine, 64-65